STUDY GUIDE TO ACCOMPANY

Nursing Research
Methods, Critical Appraisal, and Utilization
Fifth Edition

Kathleen Rose-Grippa, PhD, RN
Professor
School of Nursing
Ohio University
Athens, Ohio

Mary Jo Gorney-Moreno, PhD, RN
Associate Vice President
Academic Technology
San Jose State University
San Jose, California

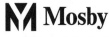 Mosby
An Affiliate of Elsevier, Inc.

St. Louis   London   Philadelphia   Sydney   Toronto

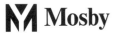

An Affiliate of Elsevier, Inc.

11830 Westline Industrial Drive
St. Louis, Missouri 63146

Study Guide to Accompany Nursing Research: Methods, Critical Appraisal, and Utilization, 5th Edition

Copyright © 2003, 1998, Mosby, Inc. All rights reserved.

NOTICE

Nursing is an ever-changing field. Standard safety precautions must be followed, but as new research and clinical experience broaden our knowledge, changes in treatment and drug therapy may become necessary or appropriate. Readers are advised to check the most current product information provided by the manufacturer of each drug to be administered to verify the recommended dose, the method and duration of administration, and contraindications. It is the responsibility of the licensed prescriber, relying on experience and knowledge of the patient, to determine dosages and the best treatment for each individual patient. Neither the publisher nor the author assumes any liability for any injury and/or damage to persons or property arising from this publication.

The Publisher

International Standard Book Number 0-323-02589-7

Executive Publisher: Barbara Nelson Cullen
Managing Editor: Lee Henderson

Printed in the United States of America

Last digit is the print number: 9 8 7 6 5 4 3 2 1

Contributors

Sharon A. Denham, DSN, RN
Associate Professor
School of Nursing
Ohio University
Athens, Ohio

Chapter 6, *Introduction to Qualitative Research*
Chapter 7, *Qualitative Approaches to Research*
Chapter 8, *Evaluating Qualitative Research*

Mary Jo Gorney-Moreno, PhD, RN
Associate Vice President
Academic Technology
San Jose State University
San Jose, California

Chapter 13, *Legal and Ethical Issues*

Kathleen Rose-Grippa, PhD, RN
Professor
School of Nursing
Ohio University
Athens, Ohio

Chapter 9, *Introduction to Quantitative Research*
Chapter 10, *Experimental and Quasiexperimental Designs*
Chapter 11, *Nonexperimental Designs*
Chapter 12, *Sampling*
Chapter 14, *Data Collection Methods*
Chapter 15, *Reliability and Validity*
Chapter 16, *Descriptive Data Analysis*
Chapter 17, *Inferential Data Analysis*
Chapter 18, *Analysis of Findings*
Chapter 19, *Evaluating Quantitative Research*
Chapter 20, *Use of Research in Practice*

Therese Snively, PhD, RN
Assistant Professor
School of Nursing
Ohio University
Athens, Ohio

Dedication

To Paul, without whom none of it would have been possible.

To Rebekah, Carolyn, Richard, Greg, Caitlin, Lydia, Sarah, Matthew, and Michael, who have taught me to make every minute count.

To my parents, Dee and Dick, for many years of support and encouragement.

To E. Pieper, for requiring a written Christmas story with no verbs.

To all of the students who have had the courage and commitment to ask a question.

Introduction

Information bombards us! The student lament used to be "I can't find any information on X." Now the cry is "What do I do with all of the information on X?" The focus shifts from finding information to thinking about how to use information. What information is worth keeping? What should be discarded? What is useful to practice? What is fluff? Where are the gaps?

Thinking about the links between information and practice is critical to the improvement of the nursing care we deliver. As each of us strengthens our individual understanding of the links between interventions and outcomes, we move the discipline's collective practice closer to being truly evidence-based. We can "know" what intervention works best in what situation.

"Helping people get better" begins with thinking. Our intent is that the activities in the study guide will help you strengthen your skills in thinking about information. The activities are designed to assist you in evaluating the research you read so you are prepared to undertake the critical analysis of all research studies. As you practice the critiquing skills addressed in this study guide, you will be strengthening your ability to make practice-based decisions grounded in nursing theory and research.

What an incredible time to be a nurse!

General Directions

1. Complete each chapter and the activities in that chapter sequentially. This study guide is designed so that you build on the knowledge gained in Chapter 1 to complete the activities in Chapter 2, and so forth. The activities are designed to give you the opportunity to apply the knowledge learned in the textbook and actually use this knowledge to solve problems, thereby gaining increased confidence that comes only from working through each chapter.

2. Follow the specific directions that precede each activity. Be certain that you have the resources needed to complete the activity before you begin that activity.

3. Do the post-test after all of the chapter's activities have been completed. The answers for the post-test items can be found on the LoBiondo-Wood and Haber web site. If in doubt, check with your instructor for the answers. If you answer 85% of the questions correctly, be confident that you have grasped the essential material presented in the chapter.

4. Clarify any questions, confusion, or concerns you may have with your instructor, or e-mail K. Rose-Grippa (grippa@ohio.edu).

5. We recommend that you read the textbook chapter first, then complete the study guide activities for that chapter.

Activity Answers Are in the Back of this Book

Answers in a workbook such as this are not "cut and dried" like answers in a math book. Many times you are asked to make a judgment call about a particular problem. If your judgment differs from that of the authors, review the criteria that you used to make your decision. Determine if you followed a logical progression of steps to reach your conclusion. If not, rework the activity. If the process you followed appears logical, and your answer remains different, remember that even experts may disagree on many of the judgment calls in nursing research. There will continue to be many "gray areas." If you average an 85% agreement with the authors, you can be sure that you are on the right track and should feel very confident about your level of expertise.

Kathleen Rose-Grippa, PhD, RN
E-mail: grippa@ohio.edu

Contents

THERESE SNIVELY

1

The Role of Research in Nursing

Introduction

One goal of this chapter in the study guide is to assist you in reviewing the material presented in Chapter 1 of the text written by LoBiondo-Wood and Haber. A second and more fundamental goal is to provide you with an opportunity to begin practicing the role of a critical consumer of research. Succeeding chapters in this workbook fine-tune your ability to evaluate research studies critically.

Learning Outcomes

On completion of this chapter, the student should be able to do the following:

- Utilize research terminology appropriately.
- Identify the research roles associated with each of the educational preparation levels of nurses.
- Identify significant events in the history of nursing research.
- Identify nursing's role in future trends in research.
- Critically analyze the significance of nursing research to own nursing role.

ACTIVITY 1

Match the term in Column B with the appropriate phrase in Column A. Each term will only be used once. This may be a good time to review the glossary.

Column A	Column B
1. _____ Systematic inquiry into possible relationships among particular phenomena	a. Critique
	b. Consumer
2. _____ One who reads critically and applies research findings in nursing practice	c. Research
3. _____ Examines the effects of nursing care on patient outcomes in a systematic process	d. Clinical research
	e. Basic research
4. _____ Critically evaluates a research report's content based on a set of criteria to evaluate the scientific merit for application	f. Research utilization
5. _____ Implementation of a scientifically sound research-based innovation into clinical practice	
6. _____ Theoretical or pure research that generates, tests, and expands theories that explain phenomena	

Check your answers with those in Appendix A, Chapter 1.

ACTIVITY 2

Listed below are specific research activities. Using the American Nurses' Association (ANA) guidelines, indicate which group of nurses has the primary responsibility for each activity. Use the abbreviations from the key provided.

Key: A = Associate degree   C = Master's degree
         B = Baccalaureate degree   D = Doctoral degree

1. _____ Design and conduct research studies.

2. _____ Identify nursing problems needing investigation.

3. _____ Assist others in applying nursing's scientific knowledge.

4. _____ Develop methods of scientific inquiry.

5. _____ Assist in data collection activities.

6. _____ Be a knowledgeable consumer of research.

7. _____ Demonstrate an awareness of the value of nursing research.

8. _____ Collaborate with an experienced researcher in proposal development, data analysis, and interpretation.

9. _____ Promote the integration of research into clinical practice.

Check your answers with those in Appendix A, Chapter 1.

ACTIVITY 3

1. Examine the four articles that are in the appendices of the LoBiondo-Wood and Haber book. What is the educational preparation of the person(s) responsible for each study? List the degrees (i.e., RN, BSN, MS, PhD, or DNSc) of each author next to the author's name. Remember, this information is usually found in the short biographical paragraph on the first page or at the end of the article.

   a. Bull, _____; Hansen, _____; and Gross, _____

   b. Cohen, _____ and Ley, _____

   c. Mahon, _____; Yarcheski, _____; and Yarcheski, _____

   d. LoBiondo-Wood, _____; Williams,_____; Kouzekanani, _____; and McGhee, _____

2. In what way does this information regarding the educational preparation of the researcher influence your thinking about the study? Before drawing any conclusions, answer the following questions:

   a. Is the first author's education preparation at the doctoral level? (Circle the correct answer.)

Appendix A	Yes No
Appendix B	Yes No
Appendix C	Yes No
Appendix D	Yes No

   The general assumption is that the first author carries the major responsibility for the research.

b. If there are other authors, is there other evidence of his or her role in the research (such as data collector) and is this congruent with ANA's prescription for roles based on educational preparation?

Appendix A

Appendix B

Appendix C

Appendix D

c.   Were any of the studies funded by external funding agencies? Write below which study, if any, received external funding. Name the agency that provided the funding. This would indicate that the research proposal had been reviewed by an external source and deemed meritorious enough to receive funding to complete the study.

Appendix A

Appendix B

Appendix C

Appendix D

Check your answers with those in Appendix A, Chapter 1.

ACTIVITY 4

Complete the following crossword puzzle as you would any other crossword puzzle. Note that if more than one word is needed in an answer, there will be no blank spaces between the two (or more) words of the name or phrase. Refer to the text for help.

Across
2. Lydia Hall's research led to the creation of this totally nurse-run health care facility.
5. Year *Clinical Practice Guidelines: Urinary Incontinence, Acute Pain Management,* and *Pressure Ulcers* were published by AHCPR. (*Numerical*)
6. Focus of nursing research between 1900 and 1950.
7. Currently there are more than ____ research centers in 32 states. (*Numerical*)
10. *Healthy People* ____ was published by the Public Health Service. (*Numerical*)
11. The 1920s saw much of this type of research published in the *American Journal of Nursing* (AJN). (2 words)
12. In 1981 the ANA published guidelines for the role of the nurse in research. What synonym for the word *research* was used in the title? (*Hint*: Check reference list.)
14. They studied aspects of thanatology, the care of dying patients, and their caretakers. (Note: Use ampersand [&] between names.)
16. Collected and analyzed data on the health status of the British Army during the Crimean War.
19. Historically, this group has been excluded from clinical research and is likely to be a major funding target in the future.
20. The research of ____ and ____ led to New York City's hiring of school nurses. (Note: use ampersand [&] between names.)
21. National Center for ____ Research established in 1986 at NIH.

Down
1. A decade of increased interest in practice-oriented research. (*Numerical*)
3. Focus of U.S. public health-funded nursing research in the 1950s. (*Abbreviate last plural word.*)
4. One of the first topics of clinically oriented research in the early half of the century.
7. First year of the decade in which the journal *Nursing Research* was first published. (*Numerical*)
8. Earliest nursing research course taught in this decade. (*Numerical*)
9. Lamb (1992) reports that a series of ____ studies demonstrated that the community-based nursing care delivery model has a positive impact on quality outcomes.
13. Researcher who conducted a classic, clinically oriented study of safety and cost savings of early hospital discharge of very-low-birth-weight infants.
15. This organization sponsored the first nursing research conference in 1967. (*Initials only*)
17. ____ report in 1923 sponsored by Rockefeller Foundation emphasized the need for nursing education to move into the university.
18. First nurse to keep systematic records of patient care (such records are critical to retrospective research). (*First initial and last name*)

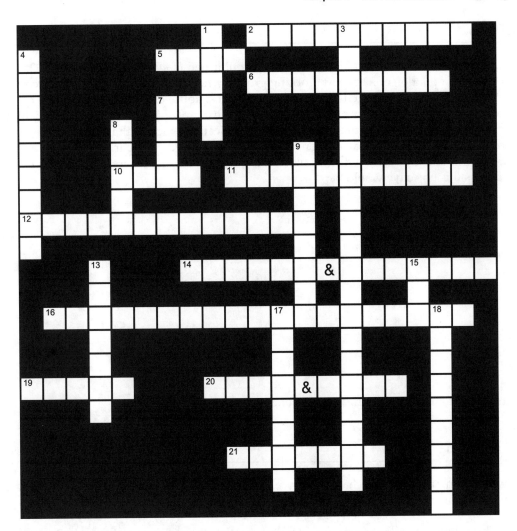

Check your answers with those in Appendix A, Chapter 1.

AHRQ's guidelines are available at their web site (http://www.ahrc.gov) or by phone at 1-800-358-9295; from outside the United States call (410) 381-3150.

ACTIVITY 5

The Department of Health and Human Services published *Healthy People 2000* in 1992. The report is a compilation of 22 expert working groups who specified many health objectives for the U.S. One of these objectives: "to reduce physical abuse directed at women by male partners to no more than 27 per 1,000 couples." One example of the way nursing is helping to achieve this objective is through studies and publications such as the 1993 *Nursing Research* article, "Physical and emotional abuse in pregnancy: a comparison of adult and teen-age women" by Parker. Other ways nursing and nurse researchers could have helped to address this objective would be:

a.

b.

c.

d.

Check your answers with those in Appendix A, Chapter 1.

ACTIVITY 6

Now that you have read the chapter, answer the following questions in your own words in a way that is meaningful to you.

1. Why is knowing about nursing research important to me as practicing nurse?

2. How will nurses produce depth in nursing science?

3. If you were asked to give testimony about your practice to the local city council, state assembly, or senate, what research information would you like to have to assist you in presenting the testimony?

Check your answers with those in Appendix A, Chapter 1.

ACTIVITY 7

Web-Based Activity

1. Go to the website: http://www.ahrc.gov/about/nrsrscix.htm.
2. Read the following:
    a. About Nurses at AHRQ
    b. Senior Scholar in Nursing
    c. Future Directions in Primary Care Research: New Special Issues for Nurses (found under Tools and Resources)
3. Under the title *Research Findings*, choose a research activity and read the report.

POST-TEST

1. Listed below are descriptions of research activities being carried out by nurses. Indicate in the space in front of each description for which of the following the action is most appropriate:

    A = An associate degree-prepared nurse
    B = A baccalaureate degree-prepared nurse
    C = A master's-prepared nurse
    D = A doctorally prepared nurse

    a. _____ Provide expert consulting to a unit that is considering changing its practice on the care of decubitus ulcers based on the results from a series of studies.

    b. _____ Take and record the blood pressures of hypertensive clients during their monthly visits to the clinic. Blood pressures are taken as part of a study on the effects of contingency contracting by a nurse researcher.

    c. _____ To understand and critically appraise research studies to discriminate whether a study is provocative or whether the findings have sufficient support to be considered for utilization.

    d. _____ Design and conduct research studies to expand nursing knowledge such as the Anderson (1993) study, *The Parenting Profile Assessment: Screening for Child Abuse.*

2. Match the terms in Column B with the appropriate phrase in Column A. Not all terms from Column B will be used.

Column A	Column B
1. _____ First nursing doctoral program began at Teacher's College, Columbia University	A. 1995 to 1999
	B. Mid- and late 19th century
2. _____ National Institute for Nursing Research authorized	C. 1992
3. _____ Nightingale studied mortality rates of British in Crimean War	D. 1924
	E. 1993
4. _____ NINR areas of special interest for these years include testing community-based nursing models	F. 1952
	G. 1900
5. _____ *Nursing Research* publication began	H. 2000

The answers to the post-test are on the textbook's web site. Please check with your instructor for these answers.

REFERENCES

Bull MJ, Hansen HE, and Gross CR (2000). A professional-patient partnership model of discharge planning with elders hospitalized with heart failure, *Appl Nurs Res* 13(1):19–28.

Cohen MZ and Ley CD (2000). Bone marrow transplantation: the battle for hope in face of fear, *Oncol Nurs Forum* 27(3):473–480.

LoBiondo-Wood G, Williams L, Kouzekanani K, and McGhee C (2000). Family adaptation to a child's transplant: pretransplant phase, *Progress in Transplantation* 10(2):81–87.

Mahon NE, Yarcheski A, and Yarcheski T (2000). Positive and negative outcomes of anger in early adolescents, *Res Nurs Health* 23:17–24.

Parker B et al. (1993). Physical and emotional abuse in pregnancy: a comparison of adult and teen-age women, *Nurs Res* 42(3):173–178.

U.S. Department of Health and Human Services (1992). *Healthy people 2000: summary report*, No. PH591–50213, Boston, Jones & Bartlett.

THERESE SNIVELY

Critical Reading Strategies: Overview of the Research Process

2

Introduction

Tools are needed for whatever task one sets out to do. Sometimes the tools are relatively simple and concrete (e.g., a pencil). Other times the tools are abstract and more difficult to describe. The tools you need to critically consider research fit into the abstract tool category. They are tools of the mind (e.g., critical thinking and critical reading tools). The following activities are designed to help you recognize and use these tools.

Learning Outcomes

On completion of this chapter, the student should be able to do the following:

- Identify the characteristics of critical thinking.
- Identify the components of critical reading.
- Use the components of critical thinking and reading on selected passages.
- Identify the format and style of quantitative versus qualitative research articles.

ACTIVITY 1

Complete each item with the appropriate word or phrase from the text.

1. Critical thinking is a(n) _____ (rational; irrational) process.

2. A noted theorist, Paul (1995), states that critical thinking is a(n) _____ (active; passive), intellectually engaging process in which the reader participates in an _____ (inner; outer) dialogue with the writer.

3. To read critically, readers must enter the point of view of someone other than themselves. The reader must enter the point of view of the _____.

4. Nursing students are first introduced to critical thinking skills through utilization of the _____ process of assessment, diagnosis, planning, intervention, and evaluation.

5. What is the minimum number of readings of a research article recommended in the text? _____

Check your answers with those in Appendix A, Chapter 2.

ACTIVITY 2

Match the term in Column B with the appropriate phrase in Column A. Terms from Column B will be used more than once.

Column A	**Column B**
1. _____ To get a general sense of the material	a. Critical thinking (CT)
2. _____ Clarify unfamiliar terms with text	b. Critical reading (CR)
3. _____ Using constructive skepticism	
4. _____ Question assumptions	
5. _____ Rational examination of ideas	
6. _____ Thinking about your own thinking	

Check your answers with those in Appendix A, Chapter 2.

ACTIVITY 3

1. The process of critical reading has four levels, or stages, of understanding. The levels are listed below in a scrambled order. Rearrange the components into the correct order.

    Scrambled order:
    Synthesis understanding
    Preliminary understanding
    Comprehensive understanding
    Analysis understanding

    Appropriate order:

    a. _____

    b. _____

    c. _____

    d. _____

2. Synthesis understanding, or putting it all together, is one of the final steps in critical reading. It can easily be broken into a series of activities that work best if completed in order. The steps are listed below in a scrambled order. Rearrange each set into the appropriate order.

    Scrambled order:
    Staple the summary to the top of copied article.
    Summarize study in own words.
    Complete one handwritten 5 x 8 card per study.
    Review the notes you have written on your copy of the article.
    Read the article for the fourth time.

    Appropriate order:

    a. _____

    b. _____

    c. _____

    d. _____

    e. _____

Check your answers with those in Appendix A, Chapter 2.

ACTIVITY 4

Determine whether the article in Appendix D (LoBiondo-Wood G, Williams L, Kouzekanani K, & McGhee C, 2000) is a quantitative or qualitative study. Utilize the following points to determine if the study you are reading is of a quantitative design. First answer *yes* or *no* for each item, then summarize your thoughts in a paragraph.

1.   Hypotheses are stated or implied in the article.   Yes   No

2.   The terms *control* and *treatment* group appear.   Yes   No

3.   The terms *survey, correlational,* or *ex post facto* are used. (*Note:* Read the glossary definitions for help in answering this question.)   Yes   No

4.   The terms *random* or *convenience* are mentioned in relation to the sample.   Yes   No

5.   Variables are measured by instruments or tools.   Yes   No

6.   Reliability and validity of instruments are discussed.   Yes   No

7.   Statistical analyses are used.   Yes   No

   Summary

Check your answers with those in Appendix A, Chapter 2.

ACTIVITY 5

You are reading the Mahon et al. (2000) article in Appendix C and find a reference to the positive outcomes of anger: "The positive outcomes of anger, such as feelings of vigor and inclination to change (Freeberg, 1982; Gaylin, 1984; Izard, 1977, 1991; Lerner, 1975; Novaco, 1976), also are clearly delineated in the theoretical literature." You are not familiar with the positive outcomes of anger, but believe that you could understand the article better if you could learn more about it. How will you quickly find out about this theory?

Check your answers with those in Appendix A, Chapter 2.

ACTIVITY 6

Web-Based Activity

Go to the website http://www.criticalthinking.org. Click on Library (found under Colleges and Universities).
   Read the following:

- A brief history of the idea of critical thinking
- Defining critical thinking
- Content is thinking: thinking is content
- Newton, Darwin, and Einstein: three distinguished questioners

POST-TEST

1. In analyzing research articles it is important to remember that the researcher may _____ (omit; vary) the steps slightly, but that the steps must still be systematically addressed.

2. To critically read a research study, the reader must have skilled reading, writing, and reasoning abilities. Use these abilities to read the following abstract, then identify concepts, clarify any unfamiliar concepts or terms, and question any assumptions or rationales presented.

> This article describes risky drug and sexual behavior and mental health characteristics in a sample of 240 homeless or drug-recovering women and their most immediate sources of social support.... Fifty-one percent of the women and 31% of their support sources had Center for Epidemiological Studies Depression Scale (CES-D) scores of 27 or greater, suggesting a high level of depressive disorders in both samples. Similarly, 76% of the women and 59% of their support sources had psychological well-being scores below a standard clinical cutoff point. These data suggest that homeless and impoverished women turn to individuals who are themselves at high risk for emotional distress and risky behaviors as their main sources of support. (Nyamathi A, Flaskerud J, and Leake B, 1997)

   a. Identify concepts.

   b.   List any unfamiliar concepts or terms that you would need to clarify.

   c.   What assumptions or rationales would you question?

3.   Quantitative and qualitative articles will vary a great deal in format and style when they appear in journals. The following statements will focus your attention on these differences and help you to distinguish between the two major types of research. Answer the following questions by inserting the correct term from the list provided. Not all terms will be used.

Used
Generate hypotheses
Statistical tests
Conducted
Test a hypothesis
Analyze themes or concepts

   a.   The primary difference between the two is that the qualitative study does not
_____ but may _____ .

   b.   An additional major difference is in the way the literature reviews are
_____ and _____ in the
study.

The answers to the post-test are in the textbook's web site. Please check with your instructor for these answers.

REFERENCES

Freeberg S (1982). Anger in adolescence, *Journal of Psychosocial Nursing and Mental Health Services* 20:29–31.

Gaylin W: *The Rage Within*, New York, 1984, Simon and Schuster.

Izard CE: *Human Emotions*, New York, 1977, Plenum Press.

Izard CE: *The Psychology of Emotions,* New York, 1991, Plenum Press.

Lerner HG: *The Dance of Anger*, New York, 1985, Harper and Row.

LoBiondo-Wood G, Williams L, Kouzekanani K, and McGhee C (2000). Family adaptation to a child's transplant: pretransplant phase, *Progress in Transplantation* 10(2):81–87.

Mahon NE, Yarcheski A, and Yarcheski T (2000). Positive and negative outcomes of anger in early adolescents, *Res Nurs Health* 23:17–24.

Novaco RW (1976). The functions and regulations of the arousal of anger, *Am Jour Psychiatry* 133:1124–1127.

Nyamathi A, Flaskerud J, and Leake B (1997). HIV-risk behaviors and mental health characteristics among homeless or drug-recovering women and their closest sources of social support, *Nurs Res* 46:133–137.

Paul RW: *Critical Thinking: How to Prepare Students for a Rapidly Changing World*, Santa Rosa, CA, 1995, Foundation of Critical Thinking.

THERESE SNIVELY

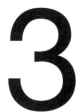

Research Problems and Hypotheses

Introduction

This chapter focuses on the problem statement and hypothesis. If done correctly, a problem statement can be very helpful to you as a consumer of nursing research because it very concisely (usually in one or two sentences) describes the essence of the research study. For the nurse who considers using the results of a given study in practice, the two primary concerns are to locate the problem statement and critique that problem statement. The hypothesis or the research questions provide the most succinct link between the underlying theoretical base and the research design. Thus, its analysis is pivotal to the analysis of the entire research study.

Learning Outcomes

On completion of this chapter, the student should be able to do the following:

- Identify terms related to the problem statement and hypothesis.
- Compare and contrast the characteristics of research problems and hypotheses.
- Differentiate between a "good" problem statement and a problem statement with limitations.
- Distinguish among each of the following:
  a. Research hypothesis
  b. Statistical hypothesis
  c. Research question
  d. Directional hypothesis
  e. Nondirectional hypothesis
- Distinguish between independent and dependent variables.
- Apply critiquing criteria to the evaluation of a problem statement in a research report.

ACTIVITY 1

Match the terms in Column B to the appropriate phrase in Column A. Not all terms from Column B will be used.

<table>
<tr><td colspan="2" align="center">**Column A**</td><td align="center">**Column B**</td></tr>
<tr><td>1. _____</td><td>An interrogative sentence or declarative statement about the relationship between two or more variables</td><td>a. Testability

b. Independent variable</td></tr>
<tr><td>2. _____</td><td>The variable that has the presumed effect on the second variable</td><td>c. Variables

d. Dependent variable</td></tr>
<tr><td>3. _____</td><td>The variable that is not manipulated</td><td>e. Problem statement</td></tr>
<tr><td>4. _____</td><td>A property of the problem that indicates it is measurable by either qualitative or quantitative methods</td><td>f. Hypothesis</td></tr>
<tr><td>5. _____</td><td>The concepts or properties that are operationalized and studied</td><td></td></tr>
</table>

Check your answers with those in Appendix A, Chapter 3.

ACTIVITY 2

A good problem statement exhibits four characteristics. Read the problem statements below and examine them to determine if each of the four criteria is present. Following each problem statement is a list representing the four criteria (a-d). Circle *yes* or *no* to indicate whether each criterion is met.

The problem statement:
  a. Clearly and unambiguously identifies the variables under consideration.
  b. Clearly expresses the variables' relationship to one another.
  c. Specifies the nature of the population being studied.
  d. Implies the possibility of empirical testing.

1. The purpose of this study was to describe the association between the marital relationship and the health of the wife with chronic fatigue and immune dysfunction syndrome (CFIDS). (Goodwin, 1997)

   Criterion a: Yes   No

   Criterion b: Yes   No

   Criterion c: Yes   No

   Criterion d: Yes   No

2. This study examined the effects of an individualized computerized testing system for baccalaureate nursing students enrolled in health assessment and obstetrics-women's health during a 3-year period. (Bloom and Trice, 1997)

    Criterion a: Yes   No

    Criterion b: Yes   No

    Criterion c: Yes   No

    Criterion d: Yes   No

3. This study was an examination of perceptions about the causes of coronary artery disease and the timeline of the disease among 105 patients hospitalized because of myocardial infarction or for coronary angiography and receiving the diagnosis of coronary artery disease. (Zerwic JJ, King KB, and Wiasowicz GS, 1997)

    Criterion a: Yes   No

    Criterion b: Yes   No

    Criterion c: Yes   No

    Criterion d: Yes   No

Check your answers with those in Appendix A, Chapter 3.

ACTIVITY 3

The ability to distinguish between independent and dependent variables is a crucial preliminary step to determine whether a research hypothesis is a succinct statement of the relationship between two variables. Identify the variables in the following examples. Decide which is the independent (presumed cause) variable and which is the dependent (presumed effect) variable.

1. The use of cathode ray terminals (CRTs) increases the incidence of birth defects.

    a. Independent variable:

    b. Dependent variable:

2. Individuals with birth defects have a higher incidence of independence-dependence conflicts than individuals without birth defects.

    a. Independent variable:

    b. Dependent variable:

3. What is the relationship between daily moderate consumption of white wine and serum cholesterol levels?

   a. Independent variable:

   b. Dependent variable:

4. Problem-oriented recording leads to more effective patient care than narrative recording.

   a. Independent variable:

   b. Dependent variable:

5. Nurses and physicians differ in the way they view the extended-role concept for nurses.

   a. Independent variable:

   b. Dependent variable:

6. The purpose of this study was to determine the extent to which sex, age, height, and weight predict selected physiologic outcomes; namely, forced expiratory volume in one second (FEV1), hemoglobin concentration, food intake, serum glucose concentration, total serum cholesterol concentration, and cancer-related weight change. (Brown, Knapp, and Radke, 1997)

   a. Independent variables:

   b. Dependent variables:

Check your answers with those in Appendix A, Chapter 3.

ACTIVITY 4

Now take each hypothesis (or research question) from Activity 3 and label it with the appropriate abbreviation from the key provided. More than one abbreviation from the key may be used to describe each item. Not all abbreviations will be used.

Key: RQ = Research question
         RP = Research problem
         DH = Directional hypothesis
         NDH = Nondirectional hypothesis
         Hr = Research hypothesis
         Ho = Statistical hypothesis

1. _____ The use of cathode ray terminals (CRTs) increases the incidence of birth defects.

2. _____ Individuals with birth defects have a higher incidence of independence-dependence conflicts than individuals without birth defects.

3. _____ What is the relationship between daily moderate consumption of white wine and serum cholesterol levels?

4. _____ Problem-oriented recording leads to more effective patient care than narrative recording.

5. _____ Nurses and physicians differ in the way they view the extended-role concept for nurses.

6. _____ The purpose of this study was to determine the extent to which sex, age, height, and weight predict selected physiologic outcomes; namely, forced expiratory volume in one second (FEV1), hemoglobin concentration, food intake, serum glucose concentration, total serum cholesterol concentration, and cancer-related weight change. (Brown, Knapp, and Radke, 1997)

Check your answers with those in Appendix A, Chapter 3.

ACTIVITY 5

The next step is to practice writing hypotheses of different types. Return to the first three of the six hypotheses/questions/problems you labeled in Activity 4. Each was labeled as a specific type of hypothesis, research question, or problem statement. Rewrite each of the first three to meet the conditions of the remaining four types of questions or hypotheses. The first problem is partially completed to provide an example.

Problem 1: The use of cathode ray terminals (CRTs) increases the incidence of birth defects.

DH   *The use of CRTs increases the incidence of birth defects.*

NDH   *The use of CRTs affects the incidence of birth defects.*

Hr   *The use of CRTs increases the incidence of birth defects.*

RQ

Ho

Problem 2: Individuals with birth defects have a higher incidence of independence-dependence conflicts than individuals without birth defects.

DH

NDH

Hr

RQ

Ho

Problem 3: What is the relationship between daily moderate consumption of white wine and serum cholesterol levels?

DH

NDH

Hr

RQ

Ho

Check your answers with those in Appendix A, Chapter 3.

ACTIVITY 6

Critique the following hypotheses. There were two hypotheses tested in this study.

1. *Hypothesis I:* There will be significant improvement in the dressing independence of cognitively impaired nursing home residents following implementation of strategies to promote independence in dressing (SPID). (Beck et al., 1997)

   a. Is the hypothesis clearly stated in a declarative form?
      Yes   No

   b. Are the independent and dependent variables identified in the statement of the hypothesis?
      Yes   No

   c. Are the variables measurable or potentially measurable?
      Yes   No

    d.   Is the hypothesis stated in such a way that it is testable?
        Yes   No

    e.   Is the hypothesis stated objectively without value-laden words?
        Yes   No

    f.   Is the direction of the relationship in the hypothesis clearly stated?
        Yes   No

    g.   Is each of the hypotheses specific to one relationship so that each hypothesis can be either supported or not supported?
        Yes   No

2. *Hypothesis II:* There will be no difference in the time required by nursing assistants to complete dressing activities with cognitively impaired residents before and after implementing strategies to promote independence in dressing (SPID). (Beck et al., 1997).

    a.   Is the hypothesis clearly stated in a declarative form?
        Yes   No

    b.   Are the independent and dependent variables identified in the statement of the hypothesis?
        Yes   No

    c.   Are the variables measurable or potentially measurable?
        Yes   No

    d.   Is the hypothesis stated in such a way that it is testable?
        Yes   No

    e.   Is the hypothesis stated objectively without value-laden words?
        Yes   No

    f.   Is the direction of the relationship in the hypothesis clearly stated?
        Yes   No

    g.   Is each of the hypotheses specific to one relationship so that each hypothesis can be either supported or not supported?
        Yes   No

ACTIVITY 7

1. You are designing a research study as part of the graduation requirements for your master's degree in nursing. In your personal time-line, you have committed 1 year (two 15-week semesters) to designing, obtaining human subjects approval, data collection, analysis, writing, and conducting the oral defense of this master's thesis. You would like to study the effect on patient outcomes on a cardiac unit based on the introduction of patient care technicians as team members to replace the primary care nursing model. The feasibility issues you will need to consider are time, availability of subjects, money, facilities and equipment, experience of the researcher, and ethical issues. For each of these issues described above, give your considered opinion as to why or why not this study would be feasible.

   a. Time

   b. Availability of subjects, money, facilities, and equipment

   c. Experience of the researcher

   d. Ethical issues

2. Another important element to consider when deciding to conduct research is to determine if this is a sufficiently significant topic to study. Would the outcomes study proposed meet the criteria to be considered significant? Answer *yes* or *no* and then give the rationale underlying your choice.

a. Yes   No

b. Rationale:

Check your answers with those in Appendix A, Chapter 3.

ACTIVITY 8

How do you determine whether a sentence is a problem statement or a hypothesis?

Check your answer with those in Appendix A, Chapter 3.

ACTIVITY 9

Web-Based Activity

Go to website: http://trochim.human.cornell.edu/kb/probform.htm. Read "Problem Formulation."

Go to website: http://www.nursing-standard.co.uk/archives/vol13-27/research.htm. Read "Historical research: process, problems and pitfalls."

Go to website: http//www.ahcpr.gov/fund/nursagnd.htm. Read nursing research agenda and identify the research questions.

POST-TEST

1. Choose the terms from the key provided that best describe items a through h. Write the appropriate abbreviation in the space provided. More than one abbreviation from the key may be used to describe each item.

    Key: RQ = Research question
             DH = Directional hypothesis
             NDH = Nondirectional hypothesis
             Hr = Research hypothesis
             Ho = Statistical hypothesis

    a. _____   There will be no change in self-rated body image among women in the three patient groups.

    b. _____   What is the relationship between organizational climate dimensions and job satisfaction of nurses in neonatal intensive care units?

    c. _____   The higher the perceived parental support, the lower the girls' general fearfulness.

d. _____ There will be a significant difference in pre-post changes in cognitive development level between undergraduate nursing students who have completed a research course and those who have not.

e. _____ The post-test mean of selected psychological variables for the experimental group will be lower than that of the control group.

f. _____ There will be no association found between the level of social support and self-care health practices.

g. _____ The educational preparation of a nurse (e.g., AA, diploma, BS) will affect his/her ability to conduct thorough patient interviews.

h. _____ What is the level of postoperative infection following the use of clean tracheotomy care?

2. Fill in the blanks in the following sentences with the appropriate word or words from the list provided. Not all the words in the list will be used.

Research hypothesis	Null hypothesis
Predicts	Validity
Statistical hypothesis	Directional hypothesis
Testing	Declarative statement
Nondirectional hypothesis	Research question

a. The hypothesis is a vehicle for _____ the _____ of the assumptions of the theoretical frame- work of a research study.

b. A hypothesis transposes the question posed by the research problem into a _____ that _____ the relationship between two or more variables.

c. _____ hypotheses are more common than _____ hypotheses in studies that utilize deductive reasoning.

d. A _____ hypothesis is also known as the _____ hypothesis.

3. Review the Mahon et al. (2000) article in Appendix C of the text.

a. Highlight the problem statement or hypothesis.

b. Is it a problem statement or hypothesis? Circle the correct answer.

c. List the variables being studied:

d. Critique the problem statement or hypothesis in the Mahon et al.(2000) article focusing on the four criteria listed below. Circle your answer.

Criterion a: Clearly and unambiguously identifies the variables under consideration.
Yes   No

Criterion b: Clearly expresses the variables' relationship to one another.
Yes   No

Criteria c: Specifies the nature of the population being studied.
Yes   No

Criterion d: Implies the possibility of empirical testing.
Yes   No

e. Has the problem been placed within the context of an appropriate theoretical framework? If the answer is yes, list the framework described in the study.

4. Review the LoBiondo-Wood et al. (2000) article in Appendix D of the text.

a. Highlight the problem statement or hypothesis.

b. Is it a problem statement or hypothesis? Circle the correct answer.

c. List the variables being studied:

d. Critique the problem statement or hypothesis in the LoBiondo-Wood et al. (2000) article focusing on the four criteria listed below. Circle the correct answer.

Criterion a: Clearly and unambiguously identifies the variables under consideration.
Yes   No

Criterion b: Clearly expresses the variables' relationship to one another.
Yes   No

Criterion c: Specifies the nature of the population being studied.
Yes   No

Criterion d: Implies the possibility of empirical testing.
Yes   No

   e.   Has the problem been placed within the context of an appropriate theoretical framework? If the answer is yes, list the framework described in the study.

The answers to the post-test are in the textbook's web site. Please check with your instructor for these answers.

REFERENCES

Beck C et al. (1997). Improving dressing behavior in cognitively impaired nursing home residents, *Nurs Res* 46:126–131.

Bloom K and Trice L (1997). The efficacy of individualized computerized testing in nursing education, *Computer Nurs* 15:82–88.

Brown J, Knapp T, and Radke K (1997). Sex, age, height, and weight as predictors of selected physiologic outcomes, *Nurs Res* 46:101–104.

Goodwin S (1997). The marital relationship and health in women with chronic fatigue and immune dysfunction syndrome: views of wives and husbands, *Nurs Res* 46:138–146.

LoBiondo-Wood G et al. (2000). Family adaptation to a child's transplant: pretransplant phase. *Progress in Transplantation* 10(2):1–8.

Mahon NE, Yarcheski A, and Yarcheski T (2000). Positive and negative outcomes of anger in early adolescents, *Res Nurs Health* 23:17–24.

Ward SE, Berry PE, and Misiewicz H (1996). Concerns about analgesics among patients and family caregivers in a hospice setting, *Res Nurs Health* 19:205–211.

Zerwic JJ, King KB, and Wiasowicz GS (1997). Perceptions of patients with cardiovascular disease about the causes of coronary artery disease, *Heart Lung* 26:92–98.

THERESE SNIVELY

4

Literature Review

Introduction

The most common usage of the phrase *review of the literature* is to refer to that section of a research study in which the researcher describes the linkage between existing knowledge and the current study. Other research-related uses of a review of the literature are as follows:

1. Developing an overall impression of what research and clinical work has been done in a given area
2. Assisting in the clarification of the research problem
3. Polishing research design ideas
4. Finding possible data collection and data analysis strategies

This chapter will help you learn more about each of these uses of the literature to provide you with the basic information needed to decide whether a researcher has thoroughly reviewed the relevant literature, and used this review to its fullest potential.

Learning Outcomes

On completion of this chapter, the student should be able to do the following:

- Identify purposes of the literature review for research and nonresearch activities.
- Identify those paragraphs in any research study that constitute the literature review.
- Distinguish between primary and secondary sources.
- Differentiate between conceptual and data-based literature.
- Evaluate the degree to which relevant concepts and variables are discussed in the literature review.
- Compare the advantages and disadvantages of CD-ROM and Internet databases with print databases.
- Critically analyze the types of information available on the world wide web (www).

ACTIVITY 1

In the sentences listed below, fill in the blanks with the appropriate word or words from the italicized terms found in the following sentence:

> The review of the literature is essential to the growth of nursing *theory, research, education*, and *practice*. In relation to these four concepts, a critical review of the literature does the following:

1. Reveals appropriate _____ questions for the discipline.

2. Provides the latest knowledge for _____.

3. Uncovers _____ findings that can lead to changes in clinical _____.

4. Uncovers new knowledge that can lead to the refinement of _____.

Check your answers with those in Appendix A, Chapter 4.

ACTIVITY 2

Listed below are examples of uses of the literature for research consumer purposes in educational and practice settings. Match the title of the research consumer in Column B with the description of activities in Column A. Some titles will be used more than once.
    You may want to review the AHRC home page (http://www.ahrc.gov) before answering this question.

Column A—Activities	Column B—Titles
1. _____ Develop ANA's social policy statement	a. Undergraduate student
2. _____ Implement research-based nursing interventions	b. Faculty
3. _____ Develop scholarly academic papers	c. Nurses in clinical setting
4. _____ Develop AHRC's practice guidelines	d. Graduate students
5. _____ Develop research proposals for master's thesis	e. Governmental agencies
6. _____ Evaluate hospital CQI programs	f. Professional nursing organizations
7. _____ Revise curricula	

Check your answers with those in Appendix A, Chapter 4.

ACTIVITY 3

What follows is a list of terms and examples describing either conceptual or data-based literature. Put a *C* if the example describes conceptual literature, or a *D* if the example describes data-based literature. Refer to Tables 4-5 and 4-7 of the text for help.

1. _____ Published quantitative and qualitative studies

2. _____ Published articles or books discussing theories or concepts

3. _____ Unpublished abstracts of research studies from research conference

4. _____ Published studies in journal describing relationships between variables

5. _____ Teel C et al.: Perspectives unifying symptom interpretation, *Image: J Nurs Schol* 29:175–181, 1997. The purpose was to introduce the symptom interpretation model (SIM) and facilitate understanding symptoms from an intrapersonal perspective. Theory derivation was used to develop SIM for understanding comparisons of known and new symptoms in a behavioral outcomes context.

6. _____ Oldham J and Howe T: The effectiveness of placebo muscle stimulation in quadriceps muscle rehabilitation: a preliminary evaluation, *Clin Effectiv Nurs* 1:25–30, 1997. The objective of this study was to evaluate the effect of placebo and "active" muscle stimulation in the rehabilitation of quadriceps muscle function in patients with osteoarthritis of the knee. All subjects were recruited from a waiting list for knee joint replacement.

Check your answers with those in Appendix A, Chapter 4.

ACTIVITY 4

Researchers who are also clinicians are interested in solving clinical problems—whether the solution is for immediate or future use. When faced with a problem in clinical practice, a clinician's common first thought is: What have others learned about this problem? The clinician usually goes first to the nursing literature to seek an answer to that question. List *five* nursing journals that publish reports or research studies that you as a clinician might study to find out more about a problem.

1.

2.

3.

4.

5.

Check your answers with those in Appendix A, Chapter 4.

ACTIVITY 5

The review of the literature is usually easy to find. In the abridged version of a research report, it is clearly labeled. Most frequently, one of the early sections of the report is labeled *Review of Literature* or *Relevant Literature* or some other comparable term. It may also be separated into a literature review section, and another section entitled *Conceptual Framework* that presents material on the theoretical or conceptual foundation for the study.

1. Examine the first two articles that are in the appendices of the text. What title is given to the literature review section?

    a. In Bull, Hansen, and Gross?

    b. In Cohen and Ley?

        (*Note:* The length of the literature review section in a journal varies. A range from two paragraphs to several paragraphs is the most common.)

2. Does the literature review uncover gaps or inconsistencies in knowledge? If yes, state in your own words what gap or inconsistency is identified. If no, simply write "No."

    a. In Bull, Hansen, and Gross?

    b. In Cohen and Ley?

3. Return to the Bull, Hansen, and Gross article. Determine how recent the articles listed in the reference section are. There should be some from within 3 to 5 years and they should portray the development of the research over time. It should read like a good detective story, where at first there may be qualitative studies that attempt to identify which variables are important to this problem or paradigm. At some point you should also see researchers progressively analyze each of the variables, gradually narrowing and defining the scope of the problem, while others continue to look at the problem qualitatively. Do you see this in the literature and reference section of the Bull, Hansen, and Gross article?

    Circle either: Yes or No

Critique the currency of the references. Write the story you see in the reference section and as described in the review of the literature.

Check your answers with those in Appendix A, Chapter 4.

ACTIVITY 6

Sometimes it is difficult to understand the distinction between primary and secondary sources of information. There is a comparison that I have always found helpful. If you are considering giving a client an injection for pain, whose report would you feel most comfortable evaluating—the report of a family member or nurse's aide (i.e., secondary source) or the actual report by the client (i.e., primary source)? As a consumer of nursing research, you will also need to evaluate the credibility of research designs and reports based in part on whether they are generated from primary or secondary sources so that you know whether the information you are reading is a first-hand report or someone else's interpretation of the material.

1. The following words or phrases describe either primary or secondary sources. Put a *P* next to those describing primary and an *S* next to those describing secondary sources.

   a. _____ Summaries of research studies

   b. _____ First-hand accounts

   c. _____ Biographies

   d. _____ Textbooks

   e. _____ Patient records

   f. _____ Reports written by the researcher

   g. _____ Dissertations or master's theses

2. The best source for primary research studies is the web.
    True   False

3. You have a computer, fast modem, web access provider, and web browser service at your home. You can now do your literature search in CINAHL OnLine without any additional cost.
    True   False

4. Information about CINAHL products and links to other nursing sources can be accessed at: http://www.cinahl.com.
    True   False

5. To use Internet Grateful Med, the user with Internet access and a MEDLARS account need only point a compatible web browser such as Netscape Navigator at the Internet Grateful Med URL: http://igm.nlm.nih.gov.
    True   False

6. Which is the best database for a search of nursing literature?
    a. MEDLINE
    b. CINAHL
    Why is one better than the other for nursing literature?

7. Print databases, such as CINAHL Print Index, must be used for literature searches of material before 1982.
    True   False

8. There is usually an extra charge for full text access to an article by fax or modem over the Internet from CINAHL (http://cinahl.com) or another provider, such as Medical Matrix (http://www.medmatrix.org/info/medlinetable.html).
    True   False

9. The Sigma Theta Tau Law Registry of Nursing Research (http://www.stti.iupui.edu/library) and the Online Journal of Knowledge Synthesis for Nursing are available on the web for free.
    True   False

Check your answers with those in Appendix A, Chapter 4.

ACTIVITY 7

Below is a selected list of references from the Bull, Hansen, and Gross article (see Appendix A in the textbook). Next to each, indicate whether the reference is conceptual (C) or data-based (D), and whether it is primary (P) or secondary (S).

Sometimes it is helpful to return to the text of the article and read the discussion of the reference; this may quickly inform you of the type of article that is referenced.

1. _____ _____   Bull MJ: Use of formal community services by elders and their family caregivers two weeks following hospital discharge, *Journal of Advanced Nursing* 19:503–508, 1994.

2. _____ _____   Donabedian A: Evaluating the quality of medical care, *Millbank Memorial Fund Quarterly* 44:194–196, 1966.

3. _____ _____   Given B, Stommel M, Collins C, King S, and Given C: Responses of elderly spouse caregivers, *Res Nurs Health* 13:77–85, 1990.

4. _____ _____   Mistriaen P, Duijnhouwe E, Wijkel D, deBont M, and Veeger A: The problems of elderly people at home one week after discharge from the acute care setting, *Journal of Advanced Nursing* 25:1233–1240, 1997.

5. _____ _____   U.S. Department of Health and Human Services, Public Health Service: *Heart failure: evaluation and care of patients with left-ventricular systolic dysfunction*, Rockville, MD, 1994, Agency for Health Care Policy Research.

Check your answers with those in Appendix A, Chapter 4.

ACTIVITY 8

Many health care professionals and consumers now use the web to search for health care information. Before going on the web , develop a set of questions that you would like to use to critique the scientific merit of health care information obtained from the web. List at least five questions.

It may be helpful to recall what you have learned about the peer-review process before journal articles are accepted for publication, and to review the critiquing criteria in the textbook.

You may also want to review http://www.widener.edu/Wolfgram-Memorial-Library/webevaluation/webeval.htm for an idea about what information is available on the web.

1.

2.

3.

4.

5.

Check your answers with those in Appendix A, Chapter 4.

ACTIVITY 9

Web-Based Activity

Go to website: http://www.cinahl.com. Explore the site and find out how much it costs to sign up for service.

Go to website: http://www.ncbi.nlm.nih.gov/entrez/query.fcgi. Work through the tutorial on Pubmed.

POST-TEST

1. Indicate whether the following are examples of primary (*P*) or secondary (*S*) sources.

   a. _____ Pell J: Cardiac rehabilitation: a review of its effectiveness, *Cor Health Care* 1:8–17, 1997. This article reviews the published literature on the effectiveness of cardiac rehabilitation in terms of improving mortality, quality of life, and employment in those with myocardial infarction and stable angina pectoris.

b. _____ Zalon M: Pain in frail, elderly women after surgery, *Image: J Nurs Schol* 29:21–26, 1997. The purpose was to describe the lived experience of post-operative pain in frail, elderly women using Colaizzi's (1978) phenomeno-logical approach.

2. Turn to the reference section in the LoBiondo-Wood et al article (see Appendix D in the textbook), which is partially reproduced below. Next to each reference indicate whether it is conceptual (*C*), or data-based (*D*), and whether it is primary (*P*), or secondary (*S*).

   a. _____ _____ Brandt PA: Clinical assessment of social support of families with handicapped children, *Compr Ped Nurs* 7:1189–1193, 1984.

   b. _____ _____ Jacono J, Hicks G, and Antonioni C: Comparison of perceived needs of family members of critically ill patients in intensive care and neonatal intensive care units, *Heart Lung* 19:33–38, 1990.

   c. _____ _____ McCubbin HI and Patterson JM: In McCubbin HI, Sussman MB, Patterson JM, eds., *Social Stress and the Family Marriage: Marriage and Family Review,* New York, NY, 1983:67–137, Harcourt Brace.

   d. _____ _____ Suddaby EC: No simple answers: ethical conflicts in pediatric heart transplantation, *J Transplant Coord* 9:266–270, 1999.

3. Fill in the correct term.

   a. There are many (advantages; disadvantages) _____ for using computer databases rather than just print databases when doing a literature search.

   b. (Primary; Secondary) _____ sources are essential for literature reviews when designing a research proposal.

   c. The consumer of research should acquire the ability to (critically evaluate a review of the literature using critiquing criteria; use primary and secondary sources to write a literature review for a research study). _____

   d. To efficiently retrieve scholarly literature the nurse must both consult the reference librarian and _____.

The answers to the post-test are in the textbook's web site. Please check with your instructor for these answers.

REFERENCES

Bull MJ, Hansen HE, and Gross CR (2000). A professional-patient partnership model of discharge planning with elders hospitalized with heart failure, *Appl Nurs Res* 13(1):19–28.

Cohen MZ and Ley CD (2000). Bone marrow transplantation: the battle for hope in the face of fear, *Oncol Nurs Forum* 27(3):473–480.

Levine JR, Young ML, and Reinhold A: *The Internet for Dummies*, Foster City, 1995, IDG Books Worldwide, Inc.

Oldham J and Howe T (1997). The effectiveness of placebo muscle stimulation in quadriceps muscle rehabilitation: a preliminary evaluation, *Clin Effectiv Nurs* 1:25–30.

Pell J (1997). Cardiac rehabilitation: a review of its effectiveness, *Cor Health Care* 1:8–17.

Pridham K (1997). Mother's help seeking as care initiated in a social context, *Image: J Nurs Schol* 29:65–70.

Teel C et al. (1997). Perspectives unifying symptom interpretation, *Image: J Nurs Schol* 29:175–181.

Zalon M (1997). Pain in frail, elderly women after surgery, *Image: J Nurs Schol* 29:21–26.

THERESE SNIVELY

Theoretical Framework

5

Introduction

It is not uncommon for the beginning consumer of research to find the theoretical part of a study to be the least favorite component. It tends to be heavily documented and is slow reading. It will not be long before you find it to be a very valuable aspect of any study. The theoretical framework of a study provides you with the opportunity to see the research problem through the eyes of the researcher. As the researcher develops and writes this section of the study, a window to his/her mind is opened. You get a glimpse of the way this particular researcher thinks about this particular problem. A critiquer's task is to listen respectfully to that person's perspective and then ask the following questions:

- How clearly do I understand the researcher's argument?
- Does the theoretical framework connect all of the pieces of the study?
- Can I see the relationship between the theoretical discussion and my clinical practice?

Most of the exercises in this chapter address the first question. Your ability to answer the second and third questions will improve as you complete the research course and as you build your clinical experiences.

Learning Objectives

On completion of this chapter, the student should be able to do the following:

- Discuss the following terms in relation to their distinguishing characteristics and value to a research study:
  a. Concept and construct
  b. Theoretical framework or theoretical rationale
  c. Conceptual definition
  d. Operational definition
  e. Variable
- Practice inductive and deductive thinking.
- Identify the major concepts in a given study.

- Trace the path of a variable from the introduction to the study through the theoretical component of given studies.
- Evaluate the relationship of a given theoretical framework to the relevant study and to clinical practice.

ACTIVITY 1

1. Jot down in your own words the defining characteristics of:

   Inductive thinking:

   Deductive thinking:

2. Play with these two kinds of thinking (i.e., inductive and deductive thinking) a bit before moving to clinical examples.

   a. Imagine you are hungry. You look around for something to eat. You find a decorative tin labeled "candy" and decide that sounds good. You open the tin and see what looks like multicolored oval beads. Sure does not look like any candy you have ever seen before, but you trust the person who would be putting things in this tin so you decide to try them. Before long you notice yourself looking for the mottled pink, orange, yellow, and black ones because these taste good. You leave the mottled yellow, white, and reddish-brown ones alone because you do not like them.

      (Inductive; Deductive) _____ thinking would best describe your activity.

   b. Sometime later you feel those old hunger pangs returning. This time that candy tin is empty. You want some more of those sweet multicolored oval beads. You start thinking, "Those beads were in the candy tin. They were sweet. There is a candy store around the corner. I bet the candy store will have these sweet beads." You walk to the candy store and discover that your thinking was correct. The candy store does have those sweet beads, and they call them jelly beans.

      (Inductive; Deductive) _____ describes your thinking style in this situation.

3. Now think about the concept of "pain." Think even more specifically about "headache pain." Picture several individuals, including yourself, when they are experiencing a headache. List your observations.

Person #1   **Person #2**   **Person #3**   **Person #4**

Look across those observations. See any similarities? Maybe a creased forehead? Rubbing temples with fingertips? Rubbing forehead? Rubbing back of neck? Grumpy? Prefer less light? Reach for the over-the-counter pain medication? Grimaces?

Could you write a general statement about "signs of headache pain"? If "yes," please do so; if "no," jot down your thinking about why you are unable to write such a general statement.

Check your answers with those in Appendix A, Chapter 5.

ACTIVITY 2

As explained in the text, concepts are the building blocks of a study. The greater the ease with which you can identify concepts the easier it will become to analyze the theoretical framework of a given study. Once you can perform this analysis, you will be able to follow the line of logic from problem to conclusions.

1. Identify the concepts in each of the following excerpts from research:

   a. "A theoretical model was developed and tested to explain the effects of learned helplessness, self-esteem, and depression on the health practices of homeless women." (Flynn, 1997)

   b. "…was to examine the relationships among illness, uncertainty, stress, coping, and emotional well-being at the time of entry into a clinical drug trial." (Wineman et al., 1996)

   c. "As part of a larger study of the impact of a social support intervention on pregnancy outcome for lower-income African-American women…" (Bolla et al., 1996)

d. "…to identify determinants of violent and nonviolent behavior among a group of vulnerable inner-city youths." (Powell, 1997)

e. "…prevalence and consequences of verbal abuse of staff nurses by physicians were examined in the context of Lazarus' stress-coping model." (Manderino and Berkey, 1997)

2. Now let's make things a bit more complex. Remember the definition of a "concept"? Sure you do! It is an abstraction. It is a term that creates an image of an idea or some notion that we humans want to share. Some concepts are more abstract than others. For example, "love" is more abstract than "table." Frequently, the terms *concept* and *construct* are used interchangeably. There is a subtle difference.

a. Which term (beauty or nursing diagnosis) is a concept? Which is a construct?

b. Think about the concept and construct in the previous question. How are they alike?

c. How are they different?

3. Now it is your turn. Choose one concept from each of the five research examples in Item #1 of this activity. Write a definition of the chosen concept. Use your own words.

a.

b.

c.

d.

e.

4. Compare your definition of the chosen concept with the definition of the same concept written by one of your peers. How close were you? Think about those similarities and differences. Assume the two of you were going to work as co-investigators on a study that addressed the chosen concept.

   a. What would you need to resolve?

   b. Look one more time at those concepts. Do any of them more closely resemble a construct?

Check your answers with those in Appendix A, Chapter 5.

ACTIVITY 3

You have identified concepts, and you have written a definition of a concept. It is highly probable that the definition you wrote had more in common with a conceptual definition than with an operational definition. Operational definitions are a bit trickier. They need to be so clear that you, the reader, have no questions about what the researcher meant by each concept.

Think about the concept of "verbal abuse." What comes to mind when you hear that term (e.g., specific words such as swearing, put-downs, sarcasm, tone of voice, loudness of voice, frequency of abuse)? Verbal abuse was defined by Manderino and Berkey (1997) as the score on the Verbal Abuse Scale (VAS). They go on to explain that the Verbal Abuse Scale is "a recently developed 65-item self-report questionnaire (Manderino and Berkey, 1994), clearly defining 11 different forms of verbal abuse, thus permitting a focused exploration of the frequency and perceived stressfulness of the various manifestations of abuse." The 11 categories of verbal abuse are: ignoring, abusive anger, condescending, blocking/diverting, trivializing, abuse disguised as a joke, accusing/blaming, judging/criticizing, sexual harassment, discounting, and threatening. Turn to the studies included in the four appendices of the textbook. Identify the conceptual and operational definitions in each of these studies. Do not expect every study to include both and do not be surprised if some definitions are implicit rather than explicit.

1. Bull, Hansen, and Gross:

2. Cohen and Ley:

3. Mahon, Yarcheski, and Yarcheski:

4. LoBiondo-Wood, Williams, Kouzekanani, and McGhee:

ACTIVITY 4

Let's take a quick look at how theory, concepts, definitions, variables, and hypotheses fit together. There will be more detail about variables and hypotheses in a later chapter, so the focus here is more on an understanding of how they are based in theory.

1. Match the terms in Column B with the appropriate definition or example in Column A. Words in bold print in Column A indicate the element to be matched to a term. Items in Column B may be used more than once.

Column A	**Column B**

a. _____ "Fatigue symptoms were measured using the Modified Fatigue Symptoms Checklist (MFSC), a list of 30 symptoms of fatigue. Scores range from zero (no fatigue symptoms) to 30 symptoms (maximum fatigue)." (Milligan, Flenniken, and Pugh, 1996)

1. Variable

2. Hypothesis

b. _____ "...**stress** and **empowerment** were used to guide this study." (Kendra, 1996)

3. Construct

4. Operational definition

c. _____ "**Serenity** is viewed as a learned, positive emotion of inner peace that can be sustained... that decreases perceived stress and improves physical and emotional health." (Roberts and Whall, 1996)

5. Concept

6. Conceptual definition

d. _____ Older (i.e., **more than 35 years old**) first-time mothers (Reese and Harkless, 1996)

e. _____ Clinical decision-making

f. _____ Quality of life

g. _____ "**Acute confusion** is a transient syndrome characterized primarily by abnormalities in attention and cognition, but disordered psychomotor behavior, sleep-wake disturbance, and autonomic nervous system disturbances are not uncommon." (Neelon et al., 1996)

h. _____ "Are there **breathing pattern changes** from test to test or from the beginning to the end of the test?" (Hopp et al., 1996)

i. _____ "The combination of **injury experience, knowledge, demographic, health beliefs, and social influence** variables will predict home hazard accessibility." (Russell and Champion, 1996)

2. This exercise allows you the opportunity to use all of the thinking you have done so far in tracing a variable from the introduction of a study through the theoretical rationale of that same study. Turn to Appendix C of the textbook and read the first part of the Mahon, Yarcheski, and Yarcheski study. Read from the beginning of the study (including the title) to the section entitled "Method." Do not read the methods section.

   a. Name the main variable in this study (read the title closely for this information):

   b. Read the next six paragraphs and summarize in one sentence per paragraph what you learned about anger.

      i.

      ii.

      iii.

      iv.

      v.

      vi.

   c. What type of reasoning is operating in this study?

   d. Were hypotheses developed for this study?

   e. Would you describe the theoretical rationale for this study as:

      _____ A theoretical framework   _____ A theory

      _____ A conceptual model   _____ None of the above

   Check your answers with those in Appendix A, Chapter 5.

ACTIVITY 5

Use the grid that follows and critique the theoretical component of the four studies found in the appendices of the text. In the grid, identify the study that satisfies that particular criterion, that is, use *B* for Bull, Hansen, and Gross, *C* for Cohen and Ley, *M* for Mahon, Yarcheski, and Yarcheski, and *L* for LoBiondo-Wood et al.

Critiquing Grid

	Well Done	OK	Needs Help	Not Applicable
1. Theoretical rationale was clearly identified. (Could I find it?)				
2. The information in the theoretical component matches what the researchers are studying.				
3. Concepts: a. Conceptual definition(s) found b. Conceptual definition(s) clear c. Operational definition(s) found d. Operational definition(s) clear				
4. Enough literature was reviewed: a. For an expert in the area. b. For a nurse with some knowledge. c. For a nurse reading outside of area of specialty or interest.				
5. The researcher's thinking: a. Can be followed from theoretical material to hypotheses or questions. b. Makes sense.				
6. Relationships among propositions clearly stated.				
7. Theory: a. Borrowed b. Concepts/data related to nursing				
8. Findings related back to theoretical base. (I can find each concept from the theory section discussed in the "Results" section of the report.)				

ACTIVITY 5

Web-Based Activity

Go to website: http://www.jcu.edu.au/soc/nursoc/html_pages/nursing_research.htm.
Click on #7, Conceptual Theoretical Frameworks. Explore the conceptual frameworks
presented.

Go to website: http://www.training.nih.gov/student/srfp/catalog/ninr.asp. Identify the
conceptual or theoretical framework for each of the research laboratories listed.

POST-TEST

1. List three reasons supporting the importance of the theoretical rationale of a study.

    a.

    b.

    c.

2. Read each statement. Decide if the statement is true or false. Mark with a *T* if the state-
    ment is true and with an *F* if the statement is false. Rewrite the false statements to make
    them true statements.

    a. _____ "Caregiving" is an example of a concept that is so clearly understood there
        is no need for it to be operationally defined in a research study.

    b. _____ The following definition is an example of a conceptual definition: "The
        Beck Dressing Performance Scale (BDPS) (Beck, 1988) was used to measure
        the major dependent variable, the level of caregiver assistance provided
        during dressing. The dressing function is broken down into 42 discrete
        component steps for males and 45 for females. A trained rater assigns each
        step of the dressing activity a score of 0 (independent) to 7 (complete
        dependence) based on the amount of assistance required to complete each
        step. Higher scores indicate greater dependence." (Beck et al., 1997)

c. _____ The words in bold in the following phrase are the name of a construct: "...define **a professional practice model (PPM)** as a system that supports registered nurse control over the delivery of nursing care and the environment in which care is delivered." (Hoffart and Woods, 1997)

d. _____ The following is an example of a conceptual definition: "Although there is no standard definition of social support, there seems to be general acceptance of some basic typologies. House, Umberson, and Landis (1988) defined social support as positive dimensions of relationships that may promote health and buffer stress." (Bolla et al., 1996)

e. _____ The following is a sketch of a concept: "...verbal abuse was defined as verbal behaviors that are perceived as humiliating, degrading, and/or disrespectful." Because verbally abusive encounters potentially can be stressful, it seemed appropriate to address this issue within the framework of a model of stress... the major tenet of this model [sic: Lazarus' transactional model of stress coping] is that stress occurs in the face of perceived demands that tax or exceed the perceived coping resources of the person." (Manderino and Berkey, 1997)

Answers to the post-test are in the textbook's web site. Please check with your instructor for these answers.

REFERENCES

Beck C et al. (1997). Improving dressing behavior in cognitively impaired nursing home residents, *Nurs Res* 46(3):126–132.

Bolla CD et al. (1996). Social support as a road map and vehicle: an analysis of data from focus group interviews with a group of African American women, *Public Health Nurs* 13(5):331–336.

Flynn L (1997). The health practices of homeless women: a causal model, *Nurs Res* 46(2):72–77.

Hoffart N and Woods CQ (1997). Elements of a nursing professional practice model, *J Prof Nurs* 12(6):354–364.

Hopp LJ et al. (1996). Incremental threshold loading in patients with chronic obstructive pulmonary disease, *Nurs Res* 45(4):196–202.

Kendra MA (1996). Perception of risk by home health care administrators and field workers, *Public Health Nurs* 13(6):386–393.

Manderino MA and Berkey N (1997). Verbal abuse of staff nurses by physicians, *J Prof Nurs* 13(1):48–55.

Milligan RA, Flenniken PM and Pugh LC (1996). Positioning intervention to minimize fatigue in breast-feeding women, *Appl Nurs Res* 9(2):67–70.

Neelon VJ et al. (1996). The Neecham confusion scale: construction, validation, and clinical testing, *Nurs Res* 45(6):324–330.

Powell KB (1997). Correlates of violent and nonviolent behavior among vulnerable inner-city youths, *Family Comm Health* 20(2):38–47.

Reese SM and Harkless G (1996). Clinical methods: divergent themes in maternal experience in women older than 35 years of age, *Appl Nurs Res* 9(3):148–153.

Roberts KT and Whall A (1996). Serenity as a goal for nursing practice, *Image: J Nurs Schol* 28(4):359–364.

Russell KM and Champion VL (1996). Health beliefs and social influence in home safety practice of mothers with preschool children, *Image: J Nurs Schol* 28(1):59–64.

Wineman NM et al. (1996). Relationships among illness uncertainty, stress, coping, and emotional well-being at entry into a clinical drug trial, *Appl Nurs Res* 9(2):53–60.

SHARON A. DENHAM

6

Introduction to Qualitative Research

Introduction

Qualitative research is a term often applied to naturalistic investigations, research that involves studying phenomena in places where it is occurring. One might say that all research is about discovery, coming to know truth, and gaining knowledge. Historically, most have viewed science from its empirical perspectives and placed great value on control, prediction, objectivity, and generalizability, terms that will be discussed more thoroughly later in this text. This received perspective has the worldview that a single reality exists and aims to identify truth in objective and replicable ways. Empirical studies are essential for investigating particular variables, but are less helpful in understanding human responses and life experiences.

Qualitative research is about understanding phenomena and finding meaning through examining the pieces that comprise the whole. Qualitative research approaches are based on a perceived perspective or holistic worldview that says there is not a single reality. Instead, reality is viewed as based upon perceptions that differ from person to person and change over time; meaning can only be truly understood if it is associated with a specific situation or context.

Five traditional approaches have commonly been used with research; four of these are qualitative methods and one is quantitative. The quantitative method is usually referred to as empirical analytical research. The qualitative nursing research methods are: grounded theory, case study, ethnography, and phenomenology. It is important to be able to identify the differences among these types of investigations.

Learning Outcomes

On completion of this chapter, the student should be able to do the following:

- Define key concepts in the philosophy of science.
- Identify assumptions underlying the received view and the perceived view of research.
- Identify the assumptions underlying a quantitative or empirical research approach.
- Identify differing assumptions underlying four qualitative research approaches (grounded theory, case study, ethnography, phenomenology).

ACTIVITY 1

Carper's (1978) seminal work has described four patterns of knowing pertinent to nursing as empirics, moral knowledge, personal knowing, and aesthetic. She described how no one way of knowing provided the entire truth, but only a perspective of the whole truth.

It is these four patterns of knowing that provide the foundation for truly understanding the diversity and complexity of nursing. Knowledge guides nursing practice! Science is an important way to derive knowledge and is more reliable than instinct or intuition. Research is about asking good questions, questions that generate knowledge. The questions researchers ask are derived from a variety of different philosophical positions.

1. In your own words, describe what Carper (1978) meant by each of the following terms:

    a. Empirical knowledge

    b. Moral knowledge

    c. Personal knowing

    d. Aesthetic knowing

2. Philosophy is based upon the ways people think about the world. One can find great extremes in worldviews or paradigms. The philosophical perspectives of the researcher influence approaches to research.

    a. Go to the web page of Beth Rodgers, PhD, professor at the University of Wisconsin, Milwaukee, philosophy and history of science at http://www.uwm.edu/~brodg/, click on "Philosopher and History." When that page opens up, then scroll down to the topic "Philosophers." Here you will see a list of names of different philosophers. Choose one name and thoroughly review the site, then write a paragraph of 5-6 sentences where you describe the main philosophical perspectives of the selected philosopher. Feel free to use a search engine to find other web sites that provide additional information about the philosopher selected.

    b. Many people view German professor Martin Heidegger (1889-1976) as a leading philosopher relevant to qualitative approaches to research. Many nurses who are qualitative researchers have used his philosophical perspectives while investigating human behaviors applicable to nursing. Go to "Ereignis" http://www.webcom. com/~paf/ereignis.html and review this web site. You may want to look for other web sites about Heidegger that provide different information. In 5-6 sentences write a paragraph that discusses some of Heidegger's philosophical perspectives.

ACTIVITY 2

In the LoBiondo-Wood and Haber (2002) text, The authors identify several terms that they suggest have meaning and are important for understanding qualitative research. Take some time to define the following terms:

    a. Epistemology

    b. Ontology

    c. Context

    d. Perceived paradigm

    e. Received paradigm

ACTIVITY 3

Review Table 6-1, Basic Beliefs of Research Paradigms, and compare the various premises of the perceived paradigm with those of the received paradigm. In 4 to 6 sentences, explain how research about pain management for cancer care might differ if you were to study this problem using these two different paradigms.

ACTIVITY 4

The author of Chapter 6 describes the philosophical foundations of four qualitative approaches to research: grounded theory, case study, phenomenology, and ethnography. Although other forms of qualitative research exist, these methods are most commonly identified in nursing research.

1. In this activity you will briefly describe each method and then state the goal or purpose for each design:

    a. Grounded theory:

b. Case study:

c. Phenomenological research:

d. Ethnographic research:

2. Choose a search engine and investigate each of the four terms online. It may be helpful to combine each of the terms with the word *nursing*. Some URLs are suggested for each term, but many others can be found. The goal of this activity is to increase your knowledge about each of the four qualitative research methods, assist you to differentiate among them, and identify ways these research methods are being used by nurses. List three new things you discover for each of the four research methods from your Internet exploration.

a. Grounded theory: Grounded Theory: Issues for Research in Nursing http://www.nursing-standard.co.uk/archives/vol12-52/research.htm

b. Case study: Using Case Study Methodology in Nursing Research http://www.nova.edu/ssss/QR/QR6-2/zucker.html
A Professional Woman Anticipating Surgery http://www.holistic-nursing.com/Case_Study1_Holistic-Nursing.asp

c. Phenomenological research: The Nursing Moment http://phenomenologyonline.com/articles/template.cfm?ID=285
Nursing Informatics http://www.nursing-informatics.com/kwantlen/wwwsites17.html

d. Ethnographic research: Ethnography Research http://tiger.coe.missouri.edu/~wang/portfolio/pages/ethnography.htm
Personal Research and Teaching http://www.bradford.ac.uk/staff/ijhodgson/pers.htm

POST-TEST

1. Identify whether each of the following beliefs reflects the perceived or the received paradigm:

    a. _____ Statistical explanation, prediction, and control

    b. _____ Neutral observer

    c. _____ Multiple realities exist

    d. _____ Objectivism valued

    e. _____ Active participant

    f. _____ Experimental

    g. _____ Dialogic

    h. _____ Time and place are important

    i. _____ One reality exists

    j. _____ Values add to understanding the phenomenon

2. Identify whether each of the following indicates an inductive or deductive approach to research:

    a. _____ Researcher uses questionnaires and measurement devices.

    b. _____ Researcher selects participants experienced with the phenomenon of interest.

    c. _____ Primarily uses an analysis process that generates a numerical summary.

    d. _____ Researcher uses an intensive approach of self in data collection.

    e. _____ Primarily uses a narrative summary for conclusions of analysis.

3. Identify which of the following descriptions fits each form of qualitative research:
    A = Grounded theory
    B = Phenomenology
    C = Case study
    D = Ethnography

    a. _____ Designed to inductively develop a theory based on observations.

b. _____ Describe patterns of behavior of people within a culture.

c. _____ Culture is a fundamental value underlying this form of research.

d. _____ This research form answers questions about meaning.

e. _____ This form of research can assist us in understanding differences and similarities.

The answers to the post-test can be found on the textbook's web site. Please check with your instructor for these answers.

REFERENCES

Bonadonna R (2002). A Professional Woman Anticipating Surgery. Retrieved December 27, 2002 from http://www.holistic-nursing.com/Case_Study1_Holistic-Nursing.asp

Carper B (1978). Fundamental patterns of knowing in nursing, *Advances in Nursing Science* 1(1):13–23.

Gernain CP (1999). Ethnography: The method. In PL Munhall and CO Boyd (eds.), *Nursing research: A qualitative perspective* (pp. 237–267). New York: National League for Nursing Press. Retrieved December 27, 2002 from http://tiger.coe.missouri.edu/~wang/portfolio/pages/ethnography.htm.

Hawley P (2000). The Nursing Moment. Retrieved December 27, 2002 from http://phenomenologyonline.com/articles/template.cfm?ID=285

Hodgson I (2001). Personal Research and Teaching. Retrieved December 27, 2002 from http://www.bradford.ac.uk/staff/ijhodgson/pers.htm.

Kaminiski J (2002). Nursing Informatics. Retrieved on December 27, 2002 from http://www.nursing-informatics.com/kwantlen/wwwsites17.html.

Sheldon L (2000). Grounded Theory: Issues for Research in Nursing. Retrieved on December 27, 2002 from http://www.nursing-standard.co.uk/archives/vol12-52/research.htm.

Zucker D (2001). Using Case Study Methodology in Nursing Research. Retrieved December 27, 2002 from http://www.nova.edu/ssss/QR/QR6-2/zucker.html.

SHARON A. DENHAM

7

Qualitative Approaches to Research

Introduction

Qualitative research continues to gain recognition as a sound method for investigating the complex human phenomena less easily explored using quantitative methods. Qualitative research methods provide ways to address both the science and art of nursing. These methods are especially well-suited to address phenomena related to health and illness of interest to nurses and nursing. Nurse researchers and investigators from other disciplines are discovering the increased value of findings obtained through qualitative studies. Nurses can be better prepared to critique the appropriateness of a research design and identify the usefulness of the study findings when the unique differences between quantitative and qualitative approaches to research are understood.

Learning Outcomes

On completion of this chapter, the student should be able to do the following:

- Distinguish the characteristics of qualitative research from those of quantitative research.
- Recognize the uses of qualitative research for nursing.
- Identify the qualitative approaches of phenomenological, grounded theory, ethnographic, and case study methods.
- Recognize appropriate use of historical methods.
- Identify research methodology emerging from nursing theory.
- Discuss significant issues that arise in conducting qualitative research in relation to such topics as ethics, criteria for judging scientific rigor, combination of research methods, and use of computer to assist data management.
- Apply the critiquing criteria to evaluate a report of qualitative research.

ACTIVITY 1

The reasons for selecting a qualitative design rather than a quantitative one are based upon the research question and the study purpose. Recognizing the different characteristics of qualitative research from those of quantitative research enables the nurse to better understand the way the study was conducted and interprets the research report findings. Clear understandings about qualitative research can also assist the nurse to apply the findings from these studies.

1. Complete the following statements related to qualitative research characteristics:

   a. Qualitative research combines the _____ and _____ natures of nursing to better understand the human experience.

   b. Qualitative research is used to study human experience and life context in _____.

   c. Life context is the matrix of human-human-environment relationships that emerge over the course of _____.

   d. Qualitative researchers study the _____ of individuals as they carry on their usual activities of daily life, which might occur at home, work, or school.

   e. The number of participants or subjects in a qualitative study is usually _____ than the number in a quantitative study.

   f. Quantitative research studies strive to eliminate extraneous variables, and qualitative studies are intended to explore _____ in order to better understand the participant experience.

   g. The choice to use either quantitative or qualitative methods is guided by the _____.

2. Match the term in Column B with the appropriate phrase in Column A. Each term will only be used once.

<table>
<tr><td colspan="2" align="center">**Column A**</td><td colspan="2" align="center">**Column B**</td></tr>
<tr><td>a.</td><td>_____ Information becomes repetitive</td><td>A.</td><td>Theoretical sampling</td></tr>
<tr><td>b.</td><td>_____ Select experiences to test ideas</td><td>B.</td><td>Emic</td></tr>
<tr><td>c.</td><td>_____ Outsider's view</td><td>C.</td><td>Etic</td></tr>
<tr><td>d.</td><td>_____ Identify personal biases about phenom-enon</td><td>D.</td><td>Data saturation</td></tr>
<tr><td></td><td></td><td>E.</td><td>Secondary sources</td></tr>
<tr><td>e.</td><td>_____ Insider's view</td><td></td><td></td></tr>
<tr><td></td><td></td><td>F.</td><td>Bracketed</td></tr>
<tr><td>f.</td><td>_____ Symbolic categories</td><td></td><td></td></tr>
<tr><td></td><td></td><td>G.</td><td>Case study method</td></tr>
<tr><td>g.</td><td>_____ Individuals willing to teach investigator about the phenomenon</td><td>H.</td><td>Grounded theory method</td></tr>
<tr><td>h.</td><td>_____ In-depth description of phenomenon</td><td>I.</td><td>Domains</td></tr>
<tr><td>i.</td><td>_____ Provide another perspective of phenom-enon</td><td>J.</td><td>Key informants</td></tr>
<tr><td>j.</td><td>_____ Inductive approach to develop theory about social processes</td><td></td><td></td></tr>
</table>

3. Five qualitative research methods are discussed in the text in relationship to five basic elements of research. Under each research element, briefly describe a key aspect of this element in relationship to each of the qualitative methods.

    a. Element 1: Identifying the phenomenon

        1. Phenomenology

        2. Grounded theory

        3. Ethnography

        4. Historical

        5. Case study

b. Element 2: Structuring the study

    1. Phenomenology

    2. Grounded theory

    3. Ethnography

    4. Historical

    5. Case study

c. Element 3: Gathering the data

    1. Phenomenology

    2. Grounded theory

    3. Ethnography

    4. Historical

    5. Case study

d. Element 4: Analyzing the data

    1. Phenomenology

    2. Grounded theory

    3. Ethnography

    4. Historical

    5. Case study

e.   Element 5: Describing the findings

   1.   Phenomenology

   2.   Grounded theory

   3.   Ethnography

   4.   Historical

   5.   Case study

4.   Briefly describe a research topic that interests you, identify the qualitative approach you would choose to study this interest, and explain why.

Check your answers with those in Appendix A, Chapter 7.

ACTIVITY 2

The literature review usually provides the background and significance for understanding a research problem. Not all qualitative research methods include literature reviews; or if they do they may tend to be much more brief than ones found in quantitative studies. The study in your textbook entitled *Bone marrow transplantation: the battle for hope in the face of fear* (2000) by Cohen and Ley has included only a brief discussion about bone marrow transplantation (Appendix B of the LoBiondo-Wood and Haber text).

   Read the literature review (p. 458) at the beginning of this study report and answer the following questions:

1.   What is the main theme of the literature review?

2. Describe the importance of this literature review in introducing the reader to bone marrow transplantation.

3. The authors chose to discuss two qualitative studies about bone marrow transplantation in the brief literature review. Give the references for these two qualitative studies. Briefly discuss the reasons for including information about these two studies.

4. Is there another topic that the authors might have included in the literature review that might have better prepared the reader to understand the importance of this study? Give your opinion and then support it with what you have learned about qualitative research.

Check your answers with those in Appendix A, Chapter 7.

ACTIVITY 3

Read the methods section of the Cohen and Ley (2000) report and answer the following questions:

1. What research method was used to conduct this research study?

2. Go to a search engine on the Internet and put in this research method, and then write two to three sentences to define this type of research.

3. Describe the sample in this study.

4. What important procedures were used to collect data in this study?

5. What methods were used during data analysis?

Check your answers with those in Appendix A, Chapter 7.

ACTIVITY 4

The theoretical underpinnings of qualitative research often make the findings directly applicable to nursing practice. Read the findings section of the Cohen and Ley (2000) report and answer the following questions.

1. How many subjects participated in this study?

2. What was the prevailing theme of the study participants?

3. In all, four themes were identified in the data. Name all of them.

4. Choose one of the four themes and briefly describe it from what you read in the findings.

Check your answers with those in Appendix A, Chapter 7.

ACTIVITY 5

Qualitative research has many uses for nursing practice. After reading the Cohen and Ley (2000) report, list some ways this research might be applicable to nursing practice.

Check your answers with those in Appendix A, Chapter 7.

ACTIVITY 6

Five qualitative methods of research are the phenomenological, grounded theory, ethnographic, case study, and historical methods.

For each characteristic listed below, indicate which method of qualitative research it describes. Use the letters from the key provided.

Key: A = Phenomenological
         B = Grounded theory
         C = Ethnographic
         D = Historical
         E = Case Study

a. _____ Uses primary and secondary sources.

b. _____ Uses "emic" and "etic" views of subjects' worlds.

c. _____ Research questions are action- or change-oriented.

d. _____ Central meanings arise from subjects' descriptions of lived experience.

e. _____ Truth is a lived experience.

f. _____ Uses theoretical sampling to analyze data.

g. _____ Studies the peculiarities and commonalities of a specific case.

h. _____ Discovers "domains" to analyze data.

i. _____ Provides insight on the past and serves as a guide to the present and future.

j. _____ Establishes fact, probability, or possibility.

k. _____ States individuals' history is a dimension of the present.

l. _____ Attempts to discover underlying social forces that shape human behavior.

m. _____ Seldom found in nursing journals.

n. _____ Interviews "key informants."

o. _____ Presents data as a synthesized chronicle.

p. _____ Focuses on describing cultural groups.

q. _____ Establishes reliability through external and internal criticism.

r. _____ Researcher "brackets" personal bias or perspective.

s. _____ Can include quantitative and/or qualitative data.

t. _____ Subjects are currently experiencing a circumstance.

u. _____ Collects remembered information from subjects.

v. _____ Involves "field work."

w. _____ Describes events from the past.

x. _____ May use photographs to describe current behavioral practices.

y. _____ Uses symbolic interaction as a theoretical base.

z. _____ Uses an inductive approach to understanding basic social processes.

ACTIVITY 7

Critical thinking is an important aspect of all research. It is important to take some time and carefully consider all aspects of the research process prior to beginning. Based on the five methods of qualitative research described in the text, answer the following questions:

a. Select a qualitative method you found especially interesting and explain the two things you find appealing about this method.

b. Identify three subject areas in which this method might be helpful in developing nursing knowledge:

1.

2.

3.

c. Choose one of these subject areas and identify a research question to be studied.

d. Describe the data collection methods you would use for this study.

e. Identify the characteristics of the study subjects, where you will locate them, how many subjects you might include and why.

f. Briefly explain an important aspect of data analysis using this qualitative method.

g. Describe how you might use the knowledge gained from this study in nursing practice.

Check your answers with those in Appendix A, Chapter 7.

POST-TEST

1. Qualitative research focuses on the whole of human experiences in naturalistic settings.
   True   False

2. External criticism in historical research refers to the authenticity of data sources.
   True   False

3. In qualitative research one would expect the number of subjects participating to be as large as those usually found in quantitative studies.
   True   False

4. The researcher is viewed as the major instrument for data collection.
   True   False

5. Qualitative studies strive to eliminate extraneous variables.
   True   False

6. To what does the term "saturation" in qualitative research refer?
   a. Data repetition
   b. Subject exhaustion
   c. Researcher exhaustion
   d. Sample size

7. Data, in qualitative research, are often collected by which of the following procedures?
   a. Questionnaires sent out to subjects
   b. Observation of subjects in naturalistic settings
   c. Interviews
   d. All are correct

8. The qualitative method that uses symbolic interaction as the theoretical base for research is known as which of the following?
   a. Phenomenology
   b. Grounded theory
   c. Ethnography
   d. Historical method

9. What is the qualitative method that attempts to construct the meaning of the lived experience of human phenomena?
    a. Phenomenology
    b. Grounded theory
    c. Ethnography
    d. Historical method

10. What is the qualitative research method most appropriate for answering the question: "What changes in nursing practice occurred after the Viet Nam War?"
    a. Phenomenology
    b. Grounded theory
    c. Ethnography
    d. Historical method

11. What qualitative research method would be most appropriate for studying the impact of culture on the health behaviors of urban Hispanic youth?
    a. Phenomenology
    b. Grounded theory
    c. Ethnography
    d. Historical method

12. Which data analysis process is not used with grounded theory methodology?
    a. Bracketing
    b. Axial coding
    c. Theoretical sampling
    d. Open coding

The answers to the post-test are on the textbook's web site. Please check with your instructor for these answers.

REFERENCES

Cohen MZ and Ley CD (2000). Bone marrow transplantation: The battle for hope in the face of fear, *Oncol Nurs Forum* 27:473–480.

SHARON A. DENHAM

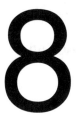

Evaluating Qualitative Research

Introduction

Qualitative research provides an opportunity to generate new knowledge about phenomena less easily studied with empirical or quantitative methods. Nurse researchers are increasingly using qualitative methods to explore holistic aspects less easily investigated with objective measures. In qualitative research the data are less likely to involve numbers and most likely will include text derived from interviews, focus groups, observation, field notes, or other methods. The data tend to be mostly narrative or written words that require content rather than statistical analysis. The important contributions being made to nursing knowledge through qualitative studies make it important for nurses to possess skills for evaluating and critiquing qualitative research reports.

Learning Outcomes

On completion of this chapter, the student should be able to do the following:

- Identify the influence of stylistic considerations on the presentation of a qualitative research report.
- Identify the criteria for critiquing a qualitative research report.
- Evaluate the strengths and weaknesses of a qualitative research report.
- Describe the applicability of the findings of a qualitative research report.
- Construct a critique of a research report.

ACTIVITY 1

The methods of presentation in qualitative research reports are different than those in quantitative studies. Nurses doing qualitative research reports are challenged to present the richness of the data within the restrictions of publication guidelines.

Review the article entitled *Bone marrow transplantation: the battle for hope in the face of fear* (2000) by Cohen and Ley to identify the ways the researchers stylistically presented the rich data (see Appendix B in the textbook). In the finding section entitled "Fear of Death and Hope for Survival," the researchers described several aspects of this experience and gave examples from the data to describe what is meant. Read through this section and find descriptive examples from the data that seem to summarize the key points.

Check your answers with those in Appendix A, Chapter 8.

ACTIVITY 2

The findings of qualitative studies describe or explain a phenomenon within a specific context. The findings are not usually intended to be generalizable to other groups, which means that persons who want to apply the findings to others have the responsibility to validate whether the findings are applicable in a different setting and with other persons or populations.

The theory described by Cohen and Ley (2000) is about fears and losses associated with the cancer condition and treatment option. The findings section compares the study findings with what is in the current literature about the topics.

1. What does the study conclude about fear in cancer survivors?

2. What does the study say about fear and anxiety associated with discharge?

3. What do the authors say about loss in cancer patients?

4. What do the authors of this study tell us about hope?

5. Qualitative research is used to examine important concepts. How does this study add to the existing body of knowledge about fears and losses?

6. Describe ways information provided in the "Discussion and Implications" section of their paper might be used by the practicing nurse who works with cancer patients.

Check your answers with those in Appendix A, Chapter 8.

ACTIVITY 3

Critiquing qualitative research enables the nurse to make sense out of the research report, build on the body of knowledge about human phenomena, and consider how knowledge might be applicable to nursing. Learning and applying a critiquing process is the first step in this process.

1. Review Box 8-1 in the textbook and answer the following. Match the activity in Column A with the qualitative research process in Column B. Some steps in the process are used more than once.

<table>
<tr><td align="center" colspan="2">Column A</td><td align="center">Column B</td></tr>
<tr><td>a.</td><td>_____ The purpose of the study is clearly stated.</td><td>A. Subject selection</td></tr>
<tr><td></td><td></td><td>B. Study method</td></tr>
<tr><td>b.</td><td>_____ Audiotaped interviews were used to collect phenomenological data.</td><td>C. Researcher perspective</td></tr>
<tr><td>c.</td><td>_____ Do the participants recognize the experience as their own?</td><td>D. Data analysis</td></tr>
<tr><td></td><td></td><td>E. Application of findings</td></tr>
<tr><td>d.</td><td>_____ Purposive sampling was used.</td><td>F. Findings description</td></tr>
<tr><td>e.</td><td>_____ Data are clearly reported in the research report.</td><td>G. Study design</td></tr>
<tr><td>f.</td><td>_____ The researcher has remained true to the findings.</td><td></td></tr>
<tr><td>g.</td><td>_____ Recommendations for future research are made.</td><td></td></tr>
<tr><td>h.</td><td>_____ The phenomenon of interest is clearly identified.</td><td></td></tr>
<tr><td>i.</td><td>_____ Participant observation was done in an ethnography.</td><td></td></tr>
</table>

2. Define the following terms:

    a. Credibility:

    b. Auditability:

    c. Fittingness:

Check your answers with those in Appendix A, Chapter 8.

ACTIVITY 4

The Schreiber, Stern, and Wilson (2000) paper entitled *Being strong: how black West-Indian Canadian women manage depression and its stigma,* in Chapter 8 of the textbook used grounded theory to discover how women from a nondominant cultural background experience and manage depression. The participants were 12 black West-Indian Canadian women who experienced depression between 1994 and 1996. The data were collected using participant observation. As you think about the design of this study, think about how you would evaluate the findings and critique the study as you address the following.

1. Carefully read the Schreiber, Stern, and Wilson (2000) article. Critique the study using the guidelines from Box 8-1 in the textbook. Read the questions in each section and discuss your ideas about the quality of paper in each of these areas.

    a. Statement of the Phenomenon of Interest

    b. Purpose

    c. Method

    d. Sampling

    e. Data Collection

    f. Data Analysis

    g. Credibility

    h. Auditability

    i. Fittingness

    j. Findings, Conclusions, Implications, and Recommendations

2. Identify two of your concerns about the study and pose them as questions that you might discuss with the investigator if you were provided with an opportunity.

Check your answers with those in Appendix A, Chapter 8.

ACTIVITY 5

Web-Based Activity

The Internet can be a valuable tool in gaining insight into any topic. Searching the term *qualitative research* can be a very helpful way to gain additional understandings about many aspects of this research approach. It is essential to identify a few quality starting points for your investigation. A couple of excellent sites to consider are Judy Norris's QualPage http://www.ualberta.ca/~jrnorris/qual.html where you can find links to many resources pertaining to qualitative studies, and Janice Morse's International Institute for Qualitative Methodology http://www.ualberta.ca/~iiqm/ where you can find information about conferences, journals, training, and international research.

    Your teacher may want to assign you particular activities from these web sites to assist you in your learning about qualitative research.

POST-TEST

1. Qualitative research findings are generalizable to other groups.
    True   False

2. Findings from qualitative research designs are viewed as less credible by nurse research-ers than those gained from quantitative studies.
    True   False

3. Auditability is an important aspect of evaluating a qualitative research report.
    True   False

4. The style of a qualitative research report differs from that of a quantitative research report.
    True   False

5. Some journal publication guidelines may impede the qualitative researcher's ability to convey the richness of the data.
    True   False

6. Journal reviewer's guidelines usually allow for the extra pages that qualitative research-ers might need to provide the detail of their rich data.
    True   False

7. _____ means that others should be able to identify the thinking, decisions, and methods used by the researcher when they conducted the research study.

8. _____ means that the study findings fit well outside the study situation.

9. _____ means that the research informants can identify the reported findings as their own experience.

10. _____ is the term usually applied to qualitative research to judge the validity and reliability of qualitative data.

The answers to the post-test can be found on the textbook's web site. Please check with your instructor for these answers.

REFERENCES

Schreiber R, Stern PN, and Wilson C (2000). Being strong: how black West-Indian Canadian women manage depression and its stigma, *Journal of Nursing Scholarship* 32(1):39–45.

KATHLEEN ROSE-GRIPPA

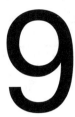

Introduction to Quantitative Research

Introduction

The term *research design* is used to describe the overall plan of a particular study. The design is the researcher's plan for answering specific research questions in the most accurate and efficient way possible. In quantitative research, the plan outlines how the hypotheses will be tested. The design ties together the present research problem, the knowledge of the past, and the implications for the future. Thus the choice of a design reflects the researcher's experience, expertise, knowledge, and biases.

Learning Outcomes

On completion of this chapter, the student should be able to do the following:

- Identify the major components of a research design.
- Identify threats to internal validity.
- Identify threats to external validity.
- State the relationship between the research design and internal and external validity.
- Critically analyze the strengths and limitations of the chosen design for a specific study.

ACTIVITY 1

Match the definition of the terms in Column A with the research design terms in Column B. Each term is used no more than once and not all terms will be used. Check the glossary for help with terms.

<table>
<tr><td colspan="2" align="center">**Column A**</td><td align="center">**Column B**</td></tr>
<tr><td>1. _____</td><td>A blueprint for conducting a research study</td><td>a. External validity</td></tr>
<tr><td></td><td></td><td>b. Internal validity</td></tr>
<tr><td>2. _____</td><td>All parts of a study follow logically from the problem statement</td><td>c. Accuracy</td></tr>
<tr><td>3. _____</td><td>Methods to keep the study conditions constant during the study</td><td>d. Research design</td></tr>
<tr><td></td><td></td><td>e. Control</td></tr>
<tr><td>4. _____</td><td>Consideration whether the study is possible and practical to conduct</td><td>f. Random sampling</td></tr>
<tr><td>5. _____</td><td>A sample of subjects similar to one another</td><td>g. Feasibility</td></tr>
<tr><td></td><td></td><td>h. Homogenous sampling</td></tr>
<tr><td>6. _____</td><td>Process to ensure every subject has an equal chance of being selected</td><td>i. Objectivity</td></tr>
<tr><td>7. _____</td><td>Degree to which a research study is consistent within itself</td><td></td></tr>
<tr><td>8. _____</td><td>Degree to which the study results can be applied to the larger population</td><td></td></tr>
</table>

Check your answers with those in Appendix A, Chapter 9.

ACTIVITY 2

For each of the following situations identify the type of threat to internal validity from the following list. Then explain the reason this is a problem, and suggest how this problem can be corrected.

History
Instrumentation
Maturation
Mortality
Selection bias
Testing

1. Nurses on a maternity unit want to study the effect of a new hospital-based teaching program on mothers' confidence in caring for their newborn infants. The researchers mail out a survey one month after discharge.

2. In a study of the results of a hypertension teaching program conducted at a senior center, the blood pressures taken by volunteers using their personal equipment were compared before and after the program.

3. A major increase in cigarette taxes occurs during a one-year follow-up study of the impact of a smoking cessation program.

4. The smoking cessation rates of an experimental group consisting of volunteers for a smoking cessation program were compared with the results of a control group of persons who wanted to quit on their own without a special program.

5. Thirty percent of the subjects dropped out of an experimental study of the effect of a job training program on employment for homeless women. Over 90% of the dropouts were single homeless women with at least two preschool children, while the majority of subjects successfully completing the program had no preschool children.

6. The researcher tested the effectiveness of a new method of teaching drug dosage and solution calculations to nursing students using a standardized calculation exam at the beginning, midpoint, and end of a 2-week course.

Check your answers with those in Appendix A, Chapter 9.

ACTIVITY 3

The term *research design* is an all-encompassing term for the overall plan to answer the research questions, including the method and specific plans to control other factors that could influence the results of the study.

To become acquainted with the major elements in the design of a study, read the study comparing two types of discharge planning by Bull, Hansen, and Gross (2000) in Appendix A in the textbook and answer the following questions:

1. What was the setting for the study?

2. Who were the subjects?

3. How was the sample selected?

4. What information was missing?

5. Was this a homogenous sample?

6. How were variables measured and constancy maintained?

7. Which group served as the control group?

Check your answers with those in Appendix A, Chapter 9.

ACTIVITY 4

Use the critiquing criteria in Chapter 9 to critique the research design of the Bull, Hansen, and Gross study in Appendix A of the textbook. (Explain your answers.)

1. Is the design appropriate?

2. Is the control consistent with the research design?

3. Think about the feasibility of this study. Is this a study that would be expected of a master's student in nursing? of a doctoral student? Explain the reasoning behind your answer.

4. Does the design logically flow from problem, framework, literature review, and hypothesis?

5. What are the threats to internal validity and how did the investigators control for each?

6. What are the threats to external validity and how did the investigators control for each?

Check your answers with those in Appendix A, Chapter 9.

ACTIVITY 5

Web-Based Activity

Assume you are thinking about submitting a proposal to NINR. You are a multi-talented researcher and are equally qualified to conduct either qualitative or quantitative research. You are curious about the number of grants awarded that would be considered quantitative or qualitative. Start at the NINR web site and describe how you could use this site to get a sense of the qualitative/quantitative ratio.

Go to www.ninr.gov. Click on each of the following in order:

Research Funding and Programs
Division of Extramural
All Funded Research Awards
FY 2001
All 2001 Awards

Review the studies that appear. Do these abstracts give you enough information to determine if the study awarded a grant was qualitative or quantitative in nature?

POST-TEST

1. Review the Mahon, Yarcheski, and Yarcheski (2000) study *Positive and negative outcomes of anger in early adolescents,* in Appendix C of the textbook. Briefly assess the major components of the research design.

   a. Use your own words to state the purpose of the study.

   b. What is the setting for the study?

   c. Who are the subjects?

   d.   How is the sample selected?

   e.   What is the research treatment?

   f.   How do the researchers attempt to control elements affecting the results of the study?

2.   Fill in the blanks by selecting from the following list of terms. Not all terms will be used.

Constancy   Mortality
Control   Internal validity
Feasibility   External validity
Selection bias   Accuracy
Reliability   History
Maturation

   a.   _____ is used to hold steady the conditions of the study.

   b.   _____ is used to describe that all aspects of a study logically follow from the problem statement.

   c.   The believability between this study and the world at large is known as _____.

   d.   The developmental, biological, or psychological processes known as _____ operate within a person over time and may influence the results of a study.

   e.   Time, subject availability, equipment, money, experience, and ethics are factors influencing the _____ of a study.

   f.   Selection bias, mortality, maturation, instrumentation, testing, and history influence the _____ of a study.

   g.   Voluntary, rather than random, assignment to an experimental or control condition creates a situation known as _____.

The answers to the post-test are in the textbook's web site. Please check with your instructor for these answers.

REFERENCES

Bull MJ, Hansen HE, and Gross CR (2000). A profession-patient partnership model of discharge planning with elders hospitalized with heart failure, *Appl Nurs Res* 13(1):19–28.

Mahon NE, Yarcheski A, and Yarcheski TJ (2000). Positive and negative outcomes of anger in early adolescents, *Res Nsg & Hlth* 23:17–24.

KATHLEEN ROSE-GRIPPA

10

Experimental and Quasiexperimental Designs

Introduction

This chapter contains exercises for two categories of design: experimental and quasiexperimental. These types of designs allow researchers to test the effects of nursing actions and make statements about cause-and-effect relationships. Therefore, they can be very helpful in testing solutions to nursing practice problems. However, a researcher chooses the design that allows a given situation or problem to be studied in the most accurate and effective way possible. Thus, not all problems are amenable to immediate study by these two types of designs. Rather, the choice of design is dependent on the development of knowledge relevant to the problem, plus the researcher's knowledge, experience, expertise, preferences, and resources.

Learning Outcomes

On completion of this chapter, the student should be able to do the following:

- Identify the components of experimental and quasiexperimental research designs.
- Compare and contrast experimental and quasiexperimental research designs.
- Critique the type of design used in experimental, quasiexperimental, and program evaluation studies.
- Critique the application potential of the findings of specific experimental and quasiexperimental studies.

ACTIVITY 1

Fill in the blank for each of the following descriptions with a term selected from the list of types of experimental and quasiexperimental designs. Each term is used only once and not all terms may be used. Consult the glossary for assistance with definition of terms.

True experiment
Solomon four-group
After-only experiment
Nonequivalent control group
After-only nonequivalent control group
Time series
Evaluation research

1. The type of design that has two groups identical to the true experimental design plus an experimental after-group and a control after-group is known as a(n) _____ design.

2. A research approach used when only one group is available to study for trends over a longer period of time is called a(n) _____ design.

3. The _____ design is also known as the post-test–only control group design in which neither the experimental group nor the control group is pretested.

4. If a researcher wants to compare results obtained from an experimental group with a control group, but was unable to conduct pretests or to randomly assign subjects to groups, the study would be known as a(n) _____ design.

5. The _____ design includes three properties: randomization, control, and manipulation.

6. When subjects are unable to be randomly assigned into experimental and control groups but are able to be pretested and post-tested, the design is known as a(n) _____ design.

Check your answers with those in Appendix A, Chapter 10.

ACTIVITY 2

Review the study by Bull, Hansen, and Gross (2000). *A professional-patient partnership model of discharge planning with elders hospitalized with heart failure* found in Appendix A of the textbook, then answer the following questions.

1. What is the name of the design used in this study?

2.   Would this design be classified as experimental or quasiexperimental? Explain.

3.   The investigators addressed two unanticipated concerns that affected internal validity.
     a.   Statistically significant difference between the two groups of caregivers.
     b.   The implementation of a CHF critical pathway in one of the hospitals.

     Which of these events would be labeled an antecedent variable? _____

     Which would be labeled an intervening variable? _____

4.   List the implications of this study for nursing practice.

Check your answers with those in Appendix A, Chapter 10.

ACTIVITY 3

The education department in a large hospital wants to test a program to educate and change nurses' attitudes regarding pain management. They have a questionnaire that measures nurses' knowledge and attitudes about pain. Your responsibility is to design a study to examine the outcome of this intervention program.

1.   You decide to use a Solomon four-group design. Complete the chart below with an X to indicate which of the four groups receive the pretest and post-test pain questionnaire and which receive the experimental teaching program.

	Pretest	Teaching	Post-Test
Group A	_____	_____	_____
Group B	_____	_____	_____
Group C	_____	_____	_____
Group D	_____	_____	_____

2.   How would you assign nurses to each of the four groups?

3.   What would you use as a pretest for the groups receiving the pretest?

4.   What is the experimental treatment?

5.   What is the outcome measure for each group?

6. Based on your reading, for what types of issues is this design particularly effective?

7. What is the major advantage for this type of design?

8. What is a disadvantage for this type of design?

Check your answers with those in Appendix A, Chapter 10.

ACTIVITY 4

For each of the following descriptions of experimental or quasiexperimental studies, identify the type of design used in the study and the advantages and disadvantages of this design.

1. The purpose of this study was to evaluate the effect of the Foster Pain Intervention (FPI) on pain and mobility. Seventy women who were scheduled for a hysterectomy completed the Preoperative Self-Efficacy Scale. The first 35 women who met the criteria were assigned to the control group, and the next 35 were assigned to the intervention group. Both groups received routine preoperative information. Those in the intervention group also received the Foster Pain Intervention information. On the first and second postoperative days the Patient Mobility and the Observer Mobility Scales were scored. (Heye, Foster, Bartlett, and Adkins, 2002)

   a. What type of design was used?

   b. What are the advantages of this design?

   c. What are the disadvantages of this design?

2. The purpose of this study was to determine the effectiveness of a thermal mattress in stabilizing and maintaining body temperature during the transport of newborns who weigh less than 1500 g. Three rectal temperature measurements of two groups of neonates were compared. Between April 1998 and October 1999 the treatment group of 100 infants was placed on a thermal mattress during transport from a referring hospital to the tertiary care center. Comparable rectal temperatures of 91 infants transported between April 1995 and March 1996 without a thermal mattress were obtained from medical records. (L'Herault, Petroff, and Jeffrey, 2001)

   a. What type of design was used? Think it through. This design is a combination of two of the designs addressed in the text.

   b. Now really put your thinking cap on and see if you can think of why this wold be a reasonable choice of design. (*Hint:* An ethical principle and standards of care are involved.)

3. The purpose of the study was to compare behavioral and interactional differences in irritable and nonirritable infants. Forty infants and their mothers were assessed every 3 weeks from the time the infants were 4 weeks old until they were 16 weeks old. (Keefe et al., 1996)

   a. What type of design was used?

   b. What are the advantages of this design?

   c. What are the disadvantages of this design?

Check your answers with those in Appendix A, Chapter 10.

ACTIVITY 5

1. You may be questioning why anyone would use a quasiexperimental design if an experimental design has the advantage of being so much stronger in detecting cause-and-effect relationships and enables the researcher to generalize the results to a wider population. In what instances might it be advantageous to use a quasiexperimental design?

2. What must the researcher do in order to generalize the findings from a quasiexperimental research study?

3. What must a clinician do before applying research findings in practice?

ACTIVITY 6

Web-Based activity

Go to www.google.com and type "quantitative research studies" in the search box. Look on the right-hand side of the screen on the dark blue bar. How many web sites were found?

Go to the tenth web site (should be the last one on the first page) and have the title "Welcome to the national center for bioethics." Whose web site is this? What is the purpose of this web site?

POST-TEST

1. Identify whether the following studies are experimental or quasiexperimental. Use the abbreviations from the key provided.

Key: E = Experimental
         Q = Quasiexperimental

   a. _____ Fifty teenage mothers are randomly assigned into an experimental parenting support group and a regular support group. Before the program and at the end of the 3-month program, mother-child interaction patterns are compared between the two groups.

   b. _____ Patients on two separate units are given a patient satisfaction with care questionnaire to complete at the end of their first hospital day and on the day of discharge. The patients on one unit receive care directed by a nurse case manager, and the patients on the other unit receive care from the usual rotation of nurses. Patient satisfaction scores are compared.

   c. _____ Students are randomly assigned to two groups. One group receives an experimental independent study program and the other receives the usual classroom instruction. Both groups receive the same post-test to evaluate learning.

   d. _____ A study was conducted to compare the effectiveness of a music relaxation program with silent relaxation on lowering blood pressure ratings. Subjects were randomly assigned into groups and blood pressures were measured before, during, and immediately after the relaxation exercises.

   e. _____ Reading and language development skills were compared between a group of children with chronic otitis media and a group of children without a history of ear problems.

2. Identify the type of experimental or quasiexperimental design for each of the following examples. Use the numbers from the key provided.

Key: 1 = After-only
         2 = After-only nonequivalent control group
         3 = True experiment
         4 = Nonequivalent control group
         5 = Time series
         6 = Solomon four-group

   a. _____ Nurses are randomly assigned to a new self-study program or the usual ECG teaching program. Knowledge of ECGs is tested before and after the program for both groups.

b. _____ Babies who tested positive on toxicology screening at birth are randomly assigned into groups to either receive routine care or to receive a special public health nurse intervention program. Health outcomes are tested and compared at 6 months.

c. _____ A school nurse clinic is set up at one school. Health care outcomes are measured at the end of a year from that school and compared with health outcomes at a comparable school that does not have a clinic.

d. _____ Diabetic patients were randomly assigned to either one of two control groups receiving routine home health care or to one of two groups with a new diabetic teaching program. Patients in one of the control groups and in one of the teaching groups took a test of diabetic knowledge as soon as they were assigned to a group. Patients in the other two groups were not pretested. All patients completed a post-test at the conclusion of the 3-week program.

e. _____ A new peer AIDS prevention program was implemented in one high school. A second high school without the program served as a control group. An AIDS knowledge test was administered at both schools before and after the program was completed.

f. _____ Trends in patients falls were summarized each week one year before and for the first year after implementation of a new hospital-based quality assurance program.

The answers to the post-test are in the textbook's web site. Please check with your instructor for these answers.

REFERENCES

Bull MJ, Hansen HE, and Gross CR (2000). A professional-patient model of discharge planning with elders hospitalized with heart failure, *Appl Nurs Res* 13(1):19–28.

Heye JL, Foster L, Bartlett MK, and Adkins S (2002). A preoperative intervention for pain reduction, improved mobility, and self-efficacy, *Appl Nurs Res* 15(3):174–183.

Keefe MR et al. (1996). A longitudinal comparison of irritable and nonirritable infants, *Nurs Res* 5:4–9.

L'Herault J, Petroff L, and Jeffrey J (2001). The effectiveness of a thermal mattress in stabilizing and maintaining body temperature during the transport of very low-birth weight newborns, *Appl Nurs Res* 14(4):210–219.

KATHLEEN ROSE-GRIPPA

11

Nonexperimental Designs

Introduction

Nonexperimental designs can provide extensive amounts of data that can help fill in the gaps found in nursing research. These designs help us clarify, see the real world, and assess relationships between variables, and they can provide clues to direct future, more controlled, research. In this way experimental and nonexperimental designs complement each other. Each provides necessary components of our lives. Nonexperimental designs allow us to discover some of the territory of nursing knowledge before trying to rearrange parts of it. It can be the basis on which knowledge is built and further refined with experimental research.

Learning Outcomes

On completion of this chapter, the student should be able to do the following:

- Identify the type of nonexperimental design used in a given study when provided the relevant sentences from the abstract or report of the research.
- Identify advantages and disadvantages of using nonexperimental designs for given problems.
- List the most appropriate type of nonexperimental design given specific research situations.
- Critique the use of nonexperimental designs for specific studies.

ACTIVITY 1

Determine an answer for each of the following items. Once you have an answer, study the diagram to find each answer. The words will always be in a straight line. They may be read up or down, left to right, right to left, or diagonally. When you find one of the words, draw a circle around it. Any single letter may be used in more than one word; however, all of the letters will not be used. There are no spaces or hyphens between the words in the puzzle; therefore, if it is a multiword answer, link the letters together as if it is all one word. While some terms will be used more than once to respond to the ten items in this activity, each term will appear only once in the puzzle.

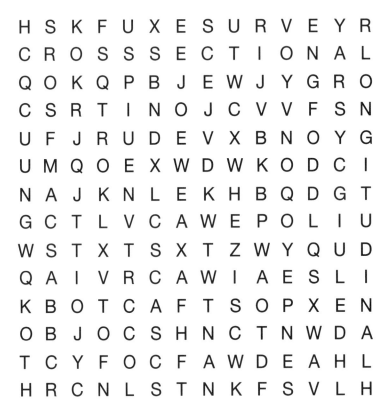

```
H  S  K  F  U  X  E  S  U  R  V  E  Y  R
C  R  O  S  S  S  E  C  T  I  O  N  A  L
Q  O  K  Q  P  B  J  E  W  J  Y  G  R  O
C  S  R  T  I  N  O  J  C  V  V  F  S  N
U  F  J  R  U  D  E  V  X  B  N  O  Y  G
U  M  Q  O  E  X  W  D  W  K  O  D  C  I
N  A  J  K  N  L  E  K  H  B  Q  D  G  T
G  C  T  L  V  C  A  W  E  P  O  L  I  U
W  S  T  X  T  S  X  T  Z  W  Y  Q  U  D
Q  A  I  V  R  C  A  W  I  A  E  S  L  I
K  B  O  T  C  A  F  T  S  O  P  X  E  N
O  B  J  O  C  S  H  N  C  T  N  W  D  A
T  C  Y  F  O  C  F  A  W  D  E  A  H  L
H  R  C  N  L  S  T  N  K  F  S  V  L  H
```

1. This type is better known for breadth of data collected than depth.
2. A major disadvantage is the length of time needed for data collection.
3. The main question is whether or not variables covary.
4. This words means *after the fact*.
5. This eliminates the confounding variable of maturation.
6. This quantifies the magnitude and direction of a relationship.
7. Collects data from the same group at several points in time.
8. Can be surprisingly accurate if the sample is representative.
9. Uses data from one point in time.
10. This is based on two or more naturally occurring groups with different conditions of the presumed independent variable.

Check your answers with those in Appendix A, Chapter 11.

ACTIVITY 2

Listed below are a series of advantages and disadvantages for various types of nonexperimental designs. For each type of design pick at least one advantage (A) and one disadvantage (D) from the list that accurately describes a quality of the design. Then insert the A or D and the appropriate number in the list below.

	Advantages	Disadvantages
Correlation studies	_____	_____
Cross-sectional	_____	_____
Ex post facto	_____	_____
Longitudinal	_____	_____
Prospective	_____	_____
Retrospective	_____	_____
Survey	_____	_____

Advantages

A1   A great deal of information can be economically obtained from a large population.
A2   Ability to assess changes in the variables of interest over time.
A3   Explores relationship between variables that are inherently not manipulable.
A4   Offers a higher level of control than a correlational study.
A5   They facilitate intelligent decision making by using objective criteria to guide process.
A6   Each subject is followed separately and serves as his/her own control.
A7   Stronger than retrospective studies because of the degree of control on extraneous variables.

Disadvantages

D1   The inability to draw a causal linkage between two variables.
D2   An alternative hypothesis could be the reason for the relationships.

D3   The researcher is unable to manipulate the variables of interest.
D4   The researcher is unable to determine a causal relationship between variables because of lack of manipulation, control, and randomization.
D5   The information obtained tends to be superficial.
D6   The researcher must know sampling techniques, questionnaire construction, interviewing, and data analysis.
D7   No randomization in sampling because studying preexisting groups.
D8   Internal validity threats, such as testing and mortality, are present.

Check your answers with those in Appendix A, Chapter 11.

ACTIVITY 3

Each of the following are excerpts from nonexperimental studies. For each example, determine the type of design used from the list provided. Not all designs are used as examples, and some designs will be used more than one time.

C   Correlation studies
CS   Cross-sectional
SD   Survey descriptive
SE   Survey exploratory
SC   Survey comparative
E   Ex post facto
L   Longitudinal
M   Methodological
MA   Metaanalysis
P   Prospective
R   Retrospective

Remember, some studies use more than one type of nonexperimental design.

1. Two groups of high-risk Medicaid-eligible mothers were compared. One group (n = 221) participated in a maternal home visitation program while the second group (n =198) did not. All mothers were interviewed in their homes using structured, face-to-face interviews. Data collection occurred once during pregnancy and once approximately one year after delivery. (Navaie-Waliser, Martin, Tessaro, Campbell, and Cross, 2001)
    Type of design:

2. One hundred-twenty (120) RNs who worked in critical care or step-down units completed the Handwashing Assessment Inventory (HAI). The consent form and the HAI were mailed to RNs who agreed to participate. A stamped, self-addressed envelope was included so the RNs could return the completed material to the investigators. (O'Boyle, Henly, and Duckett, 2001)
    Type of design:

3. Kindergarten children's knowledge and perceptions of alcohol, tobacco, and other drugs (ATODs) were assessed. Children from three elementary schools were interviewed about their knowledge, feelings, and attitudes toward ATODs using the Child Drug Awareness Inventory. (Hahn, Hall, Rayens, Burt, Corley, and Sheffel, 2000)
    Type of design:

4. The level of depressive symptoms experienced by women was measured in association with resource availability, exposure to risk factors, and intrinsic strength factors. Three questionnaires were completed by 315 women of Mexican descent living in an urban community in northern California. (Heilemann, Lee, and Kury, 2002)
    Type of design:

5. "The purpose of this study was to examine the health behaviors of nursing students as they entered and again as they completed their baccalaureate nursing education to see what lifestyle changes occurred as students were exposed to a healthcare curriculum." The procedure followed was that of the Health Promoting Lifestyle Profile, a 48-item instrument administered to students during the first and again during the last semester of their nursing program. (Riordan and Washburn, 1997)
    Type of design:

6. "Twenty-three items were initially developed for the Atkins Osteoporosis Risk Assessment Tool (ORAT) after a thorough examination of the literature. These items were reviewed for relevance to the domain of content by a panel of eight experts using Lynn's (1986) two-stage process for content validation. (Wynd and Schaefer, 2002)
    Type of design:

Check your answers with those in Appendix A, Chapter 11.

ACTIVITY 4

Use the critiquing criteria from the chapter to analyze the following excerpt from a study. In a 1997 article by Mohr, her objective was: "This study is the context portion of a larger study that described the experience of 30 nurses in Texas, USA, who worked in for-profit psychiatric hospitals during a documented period of corporate deviance. The objective of the contextual portion was to describe the major findings in 1991–1992 of investigating agencies that probed the scandal." The sample consisted of more than 1,240 pages and 40 hours of corporate records obtained under subpoena, in addition to written and oral testimony before the USA House Select Committee on Children, Youth, and Families.

1. Type of design:

The findings were four themes: insurance games, dumping patients, patient abuse, and playing with the language.

The conclusions "Organizational deviance may become more widespread in profit-driven systems of care. Lobbying for whistleblower protection, collective advocacy, and creative educational reforms are used" are presented in the frontpiece of the article. However, under the "Discussion and Recommendations" section, the author states: "As suggested by social scientists, research can serve as the basis for reflection, critique and action... For example, because nurses are professionals who have a special contract with the public and are concerned with health teaching and promotion, they might implement counter-hegemonic activity by collective advocacy and criticizing information distortion."

2. Does the research go beyond the relational parameters of the findings and erroneously infer cause-and-effect relationships between the variables?
Circle: Yes   No   (If yes, explain below.)

Check your answers with those in Appendix A, Chapter 11.

ACTIVITY 5

Review the Critical Thinking Decision Path: Nonexperimental Design Choice found in the textbook (p. 223). If you wanted to test a relationship between two variables in the past such as the incidence of reported back injuries of nurses working in a newborn nursery compared to that of nurses working in long-term care, which design would you use?

Check your answers with those in Appendix A, Chapter 11.

ACTIVITY 6

Web-Based Activity

Go to www.cdc.gov. Click on the Guidelines for Hand Hygiene in Healthcare Settings (either on the front door as a "Spotlight" or use the "Health Topics A-Z" and click on "Hand Hygiene in Healthcare Settings." Click on Fact Sheet and go to the tenth bulleted statement. Read this paragraph. Would studies using a nonexperimental design be useful in addressing these performance indicators?

POST-TEST

Choose from among the following words to complete the post-test. Each word may only be used one time; however, this list duplicates some words because they appear in more than one answer.

Retrospective	Longitudinal	Survey	Descriptive
Exploratory	Interrelational	Correlational	Ex post facto
Retrospective	Cross sectional	Retrospective	Prospective
Cross sectional	Longitudinal	Prospective	Comparative
Relationship-differences			

1. _____ is the broadest category of nonexperimental design.

2. The category from item #1 can be further classified as _____ ,
    _____ , and _____ .

3. The second major category of nonexperimental design according to LoBiondo-Wood and
    Haber includes _____ studies.

4. The researcher is using _____ design when examining the
    relationship between two or more variables.

5. _____ designs have many similarities to quasiexperimental
    designs.

6. _____ design used in epidemiological work is similar to ex
    post facto.

7. LoBiondo-Woods and Haber discuss the following *three* types of developmental studies:

    a.

    b.

    c.

8. _____ studies collect data at one point in time while
    _____ collects data from the same group at different points
    in time.

9. A(n) _____ study looks at presumed causes and moves
    forward in time to presumed effects.

10. The researcher is using a(n) _____ design if he/she is
    trying to link present events to events that have occurred in the past.

11. The following is an excerpt from a nonexperimental study. Determine the type of design
    used and insert its name in the space provided. Remember, some studies use more than
    one type of nonexperimental design.

    "This empirical study explored the attitudes and participation of registered nurses
    (RNs) in New South Wales (NSW), Australia in continuing professional education... A
    25-item questionnaire was developed and mailed to a random sample of 500 RNs
    currently licensed to practice within NSW. Respondent anonymity was assured by
    having the Nurses Registration Board generate the random sample and undertake the
    mailing." (Kersaitis, 1997)

    Type of design:

12. Review the Mahon, Yarcheski, and Yarcheski (2000) article in Appendix C of the textbook. Answer the following questions based on this article.

   a. Type of design

       Variables being studied

   Name one advantage and one disadvantage of this design in relation to this specific study.

   b. Advantage

   c. Disadvantage

   d. Does the researcher present the findings in a manner that is incongruent with the utilized design?

   e. Does the research go beyond the relational parameters of the findings and erroneously infer cause-and-effect relationships between the variables?

   f. How does the author deal with the limitations of the study?

The answers to the post-test are in the textbook's web site. Please check with your instructor for these answers.

REFERENCES

Hahn EJ, Hall LA, Rayens MK, Burt AV, Corley D, and Sheffel, KL (2000). Kindergarten children's knowledge and perceptions of alcohol, tobacco, and other drugs, *Jour Schl Health* 70(2):51–55.

Heilemann MV, Lee KA, and Kury FS (2002). Strengths and vulnerabilities of women of Mexican descent in relation to depressive symptoms, *Nurs Res* 51(3):175–182.

Kersaitis C (1997). Attitudes and participation of registered nurses in continuing professional education in New South Wales, Australia, *J Contin Educ Nurs* 28(3):135–139.

Mahon NE, Yarcheski A, and Yarcheski TJ (2000). Positive and negative outcomes of anger in early adolescents, *Res Nurs Health* 23:17–24.

McGown A and Whitbread J (1996). Out of control! The most effective way to help the binge-eating patient, *J Psychosoc Nurs* 34:30–37.

Mohr WK (1997). Outcomes of corporate greed, *Image: J Nurs Schol* 29:39–45.

Navaie-Waliser M, Martin SL, Tessaro I, Campbell MK, and Cross AW (2001). Social support and psychological functioning among high-risk mothers: The impact of Baby Love Maternal Outreach Worker Program, *Public Health Nursing* 17(4):280–291.

O'Boyle CA, Henly SJ, and Duckett LJ (2001). Nurses' motivation to wash their hands: A standardized measurement approach, *Appl Nurs Res* 14(3):136–145.

Riordan J and Washburn J (1997). Comparison of baccalaureate student lifestyle health behaviors entering and completing the nursing program, *J Nurs Educ* 36:262–265.

Wynd CA, and Schaefer MA (2002). The osteoporosis risk assessment tool: Establishing content validity through a panel of experts, *Appl Nurs Res* 16(2):184–188.

KATHLEEN ROSE-GRIPPA

12

Sampling

Introduction

Sampling consists of choosing the elements to be used in answering the research question. The ideal sampling strategy is one in which the elements truly represent the population while controlling for any source of bias. Reality modulates the ideal. Considerations of efficiency, practicality, ethics, and availability of subjects frequently alter the ideal sampling strategy for a given study.

Learning Outcomes

On completion of this chapter, the student should be able to do the following:

- Identify the advantages and disadvantages of the following sampling strategies:
    a. Convenience
    b. Quota
    c. Purposive
    d. Simple random
    e. Stratified random
    f. Cluster
    g. Systematic
- Distinguish between probability and nonprobability sampling strategies.
- Identify the sampling strategy used in study examples.
- Evaluate the congruence between the sample used and population of interest.
- Critique the sampling component of a study.

ACTIVITY 1

Identify the category of sampling for each of the following sampling strategies. Use the abbreviations from the key provided.

Key: P = Probability sampling
      N = Nonprobability sampling

1. _____ Simple random sampling

2. _____ Purposive sampling

3. _____ Cluster sampling

4. _____ Quota sampling

5. _____ Convenience sampling

6. _____ Systematic sampling

7. _____ Stratified random sampling

Check your answers with those in Appendix A, Chapter 12.

ACTIVITY 2

For each of the following examples of studies, identify the sampling strategy used from the following list. Write the letter that corresponds to the strategy in the space preceding the sampling description. Check the glossary for definition of terms.

a. Convenience sampling
b. Quota sampling
c. Purposive sampling
d. Simple random sampling
e. Stratified random sampling
f. Systematic sampling

1. _____ The sample for the study of critical thinking behavior of undergraduate baccalaureate nursing students consisted of students enrolled in junior- and senior-level courses in three schools of nursing. In each program, students were invited to participate until a total sample representing 10% of the junior-level students and 10% of the senior-level students was obtained.

2. _____ Every eighth person on the diabetic clinic patient roster was asked to participate in the study. A table of random numbers was used to select the beginning of the sampling within the first sampling interval.

3. _____ Using a table of random numbers, the sample of 50 subjects was selected from the list of all mothers giving birth in the county during the first 6 months of the year.

4. _____ The sample was selected from residents of eight nursing homes in Arkansas and consisted of cognitively impaired persons with no physical impairments or other psychiatric illness. (Beck et al., 1997)

5. _____ The sample consisted of 23 chronic pain patients participating in a multimodal pain rehabilitation program. (Vines et al., 1996)

6. _____ To study educational opportunities for nurses from various ethnic groups, a list of all nurses in the state of California was sorted by ethnicity. The sample consisted of 10% of the nurses in each ethnic group, selected according to a table of random numbers.

Check your answers with those in Appendix A, Chapter 12.

ACTIVITY 3

1. Refer to the study by Mahon, Yarcheski, and Yarcheski (2000) in Appendix C of your textbook.

   a. Was the sample adequately described?
      Yes   No

   b. Do the sample characteristics correspond to the larger population?
      Yes   No   Maybe

   c. Is this a probability or nonprobability sample?

   d. Is the sample size appropriate?
      Yes   No   Unsure

2. List one advantage of using a convenience sample in this study.

3. List one disadvantage of using a convenience sample.

Check your answers with those in Appendix A, Chapter 12.

ACTIVITY 4

Using the critical thinking decision path (page 254 of the textbook), label the following statements true or false.

1. _____ Nonprobability sampling is associated with less generalizability to the larger population.

2. _____ Convenience sampling limits generalizability of findings largely because of the self-selection of subjects.

3. _____ Nonprobability sampling strategies are more time-consuming than probability strategies.

4. _____ Random sampling has the greatest risk of bias and is moderately representative.

5. _____ The easier the sampling strategy the greater the risk of bias, and as sampling becomes easier to implement, the risk of bias and limited representativeness of the population increases.

6. _____ Purposive sampling produces the least generalizable sample of the sampling strategies listed.

Check your answers with those in Appendix A, Chapter 12.

ACTIVITY 5

Review the following excerpt from a study. Using the critiquing criteria listed in Chapter 12, page 259, critique the sampling process used in this study.

"The sample includes 20,743 students ages 12 to 21 (M = 16.2, SD = 1.7). The sample was 50.5% male. Students in the sample self-identified as Black (23.2%), White (61.6%), Asian (7.7%), American Indian (3.6%), and as members of other races (9.5%). Students were allowed to indicate membership in multiple categories. Hispanic ethnicity reported by 17.0% of the sample. The majority of the sample (57.3%) reported living in a partly rural, as opposed to an urban area. About 40% of the sample reported ever having sexual intercourse. Of those with sexual experience, 6% reported at least one diagnosis of gonorrhea, Chlamydia, syphilis, genital herpes, genital warts, HIV, or trichomoniasis. Of the sexually experienced females, 19.9% reported ever being pregnant. (Crosby & Lawrence, 2000)

1. Have the sample characteristics been completely described? (Explain your answer.)

2. Can the parameters of the study population be inferred from the description of the sample?

3. To what extent is the sample representative of the population as defined?

4. Are criteria for eligibility in the sample specifically identified?

5. Have sample delimitations been established? (Explain your answer.)

6. Would it be possible to replicate the study sample? (Explain your answer.)

7. How was the sample selected? Is the method of sample selection appropriate?

8. What kind of bias, if any, is introduced by this method?

9. Is the sample size appropriate? How is it substantiated?

10. Are there indications that rights of subjects have been ensured? (Explain your answer.)

11. Does the researcher identify the limitations in generalizability of the findings from the sample to the population? Are they appropriate?

12. Does the researcher indicate how replication of the study with other samples would provide increased support for the findings?

Check your answers with those in Appendix A, Chapter 12.

ACTIVITY 6

Web-Based Activity

Go to the US Census web site www.census.gov. Scroll to the bottom of the front door. Click on "Subjects A to Z". Click on "P" and scroll to "population." Go to "Basic Facts." Enter in the search boxes "Population, Age, & Sex" and "US by State" This should bring you to a chart that lists population data. Look at the column headed "Males to 100 Females." Look at the number of males to 100 females in the state where you live and in two other states.

Now go back to Activity 5. Would the sample in this study be considered representative in terms of gender?

POST-TEST

Complete the sentences below.

1. Sampling strategies are grouped into two categories: _____ sampling and _____ sampling.

2. _____ sampling is the use of the most readily accessible persons or objects as subjects in a study.

3. Advantages of _____ sampling are low bias and maximal representativeness, but the disadvantage is the labor in drawing a sample.

4. A(n) _____ can be used to select an unbiased sample or unbiased assignment of subjects to treatment groups.

5. A(n) _____ sample is one whose key characteristics closely approximate those of the population.

6. _____ criteria are used to select the sample from all possible units and _____ may be used to restrict the population to a homogeneous group of subjects.

7. Types of nonprobability sampling include _____, _____, and _____ sampling.

8. Successive random sampling of units that progress from large to small and meet sample eligibility criteria is known as _____ sampling.

9. In certain qualitative studies, subjects are added to the sample until _____ occurs (new data no longer emerge during data collection).

10. A statistical technique known as _____ may be used to determine sample size in quantitative studies.

The answers to the post-test are in the textbook's web site. Please check with your instructor for these answers.

REFERENCES

Beck C et al. (1997). Improving dressing behavior in cognitively impaired nursing home residents, *Nurs Res* 46:126–131.

Bull MJ, Hansen HE, and Gross CR (2000). A professional-patient partnership model of discharge planning with elders hospitalized with heart failure, *Appl Nurs Res* 13(1):19–28.

Crosby RA and St. Lawrence J (2000). Adolescents' use of school-based health clinics for reproductive health services: Data from the National Longitudinal Study of Adolescent Health, *Jour Schl Health* 70(1):22–27.

Mahon NE, Yarcheski A, and Yarcheski TJ (2000). Positive and negative outcomes of anger in early adolescents, *Res in Nursing & Hlth* 23:17–24.

Vines SW et al. (1996). Effects of a multimodal pain rehabilitation program: a pilot study, *Rehab Nurs* 21:25–30.

MARY JO GORNEY-MORENO

13

Legal and Ethical Issues

Introduction

Patient advocacy is one of the primary roles of a professional nurse. Nowhere is this more necessary than in the field of research. The nurse must be the client's advocate, whether acting as the researcher, a participant in data gathering, or a provider of care for research subjects. A multitude of legal and ethical issues exist in research; nurses must be aware of, assess, and evaluate these issues. Nurses need to be knowledgeable about the purpose and functions of Institutional Review Boards and the federal regulations on which they are based.

Learning Outcomes

On completion of this chapter, the student should be able to do the following:

- Identify the essential elements of an informed consent form.
- Describe the Institutional Review Board's role in the research review process.
- Describe the nurse's role as patient advocate in research situations.
- Critique the ethical aspects of a research study.

ACTIVITY 1

Fill in the blanks with the correct term from the following list:

Expedited review
Nursing research committee
Justice
Unethical research study
Institutional Review Board

1. _____ reviews proposals for scientific merit and congruence with the institutional policies and missions.

2. The idea that human subjects should be treated fairly and no benefit to which a person is entitled should be denied is called _____.

3. A study of existing data that is of minimal risk may be a candidate for a(n) _____.

4. The U.S. Public Health Service studied untreated syphilis on black sharecroppers in Tuskegee and withheld penicillin treatment even after penicillin was commonly available. This was considered a(n) _____.

5. _____ reviews research proposals to assure protection of the rights of human subjects.

Check your answers with those in Appendix A, Chapter 13.

ACTIVITY 2

List the *three* ethical principles relevant to the conduct of research involving human subjects.

1.

2.

3.

Check your answers with those in Appendix A, Chapter 13.

ACTIVITY 3

Review the articles in Appendices A-D of the text. For each article, describe how informed consent was obtained and how the author described obtaining permission from the Institutional Review Board (IRB).

1.   Appendix A

2.   Appendix B

3.   Appendix C

4.   Appendix D

Check your answers with those in Appendix A, Chapter 13.

ACTIVITY 4

1.   Identify *at least four* groups of subjects who are vulnerable or have diminished autonomy.

   a.

   b.

   c.

   d.

2. Identify the vulnerable populations, if any, that were included in the studies found in Appendices A –D of the text.

   a.

   b.

   c.

   d.

3. Read the following study excerpts as if you are a nurse member of an IRB. Do you see any conditions that might require special circumstances? If yes, list them below.

   a. "The study examined the effect of individualized computerized testing system for baccalaureate nursing students enrolled in health assessment and obstetrics/ women's health during a 3-year period. One hundred twenty-seven students participated in the study. The testing software, Pedagogue TM, was used to generate the computer test, and the students took all quizzes on-line. The mean score on computer tests in both courses were as good as, or better than previous scores on paper-pencil forms of the tests (p<.05)." (Bloom and Trice, 1997)

      Special circumstances?

   b. "Inner-city male adolescents in jail in New York City (N = 427) were interviewed to examine correlates of cocaine or crack use. Twenty-three percent had used cocaine or crack in the month before arrest and 32% reported lifetime use. Substantial rates of robbery, murder, other violent crime, weapons possession, and drug dealing were found. However, type of crime, including violent crime, was not related either to cocaine/crack use or to drug dealing. Current cocaine/crack users were more likely to use alcohol, marijuana, and intranasal heroin; to have multiple previous arrests; to be out of school; to be psychologically distressed; to have been sexually molested as a child; to have substance-abusing parents; and to have cocaine/crack-using friends. They were also more likely to have frequent sex with girls, to be gay or bisexual, and to engage in anal intercourse. The findings should be considered in developing more effective drug abuse prevention and treatment interventions, and HIV prevention and education for incarcerated at-risk adolescents." (Kang, Magura, and Shapiro, 1994)

      Special circumstances?

Check your answers with those in Appendix A, Chapter 13.

ACTIVITY 5

What is the composition of the IRB at your college or hospital? List the professions of the members.

Check your answers with those in Appendix A, Chapter 13.

ACTIVITY 6

In a discussion about the lack of agreement on what constitutes or does not constitute scientific misconduct, Hansen and Hansen (1995) have posed several questions to consider. The three questions that are most likely to be of concern to research consumers are listed below. For each, write your opinion below the question.

1. "Have you ever gotten a suggestion or idea for your research from a verbal comment (either in a lecture or directly to you) that you did not acknowledge in a later written report of the research?"

2. "Have you ever paraphrased a statement made by someone else without identifying the source?"

3. "Would you provide free access to your raw data to any researcher asking to use it after you have published your results?"

Check your answers with those in Appendix A, Chapter 13.

ACTIVITY 7

It is 1942, and you are the first doctorally prepared nurse at your hospital. You are approached by Sister Elizabeth Kinney to show the doctors that her treatment for spasms (i.e., paralysis of poliomyelitis) is the right way to treat patients. How would you respond to her? What would be your ethical concerns related to this research? (*Note:* A summary of Sister Kinney's methods and ideas follows.)

It may be helpful to read the fascinating article describing Kinney's life and ideas in *Image: Journal of Nursing Scholarship* First Quarter, pp. 83–88, 1997.

By age 23, Elizabeth was an established bush nurse. She delivered babies and cared for the sick… in 1911, she encountered a young girl in constant pain, muscular pain that increased severely when touched. The child's legs were contracted in twisted positions, and her back and neck were misaligned. Confused by this condition, Nurse Elizabeth telegrammed Dr. McDonnell for advice. The return message stated: Infantile paralysis. No known treatment. Do the best you can with the symptoms presenting themselves. (Kinney and Ostenso, 1943; Morris, 1972; Oppewal, 1997)

Relying on keen observation, caring concern, and past knowledge from studying human anatomy, Elizabeth experimented to relieve the child's pain. She had never read or heard of a medical treatment for infantile paralysis, or poliomyelitis, as it was later called. Fearful that contractures and deformities would permanently result unless the child's muscles relaxed, she tried applying heated salt placed in a bag and a linseed meal poultice. Both were too heavy. However, the child did respond to heat from a wool blanket torn into strips then placed in boiling water and wrung dry. Upon awakening from a relaxed sleep, the child said, "I want them rags that wells my legs!" (Kinney and Ostenso, 1943)

A year elapsed before Elizabeth discussed this first, and five other cases with Dr. McDonnell. He was surprised to learn that none of her patients developed deformities. The orthodox medical treatment at that time was to immobilize the affected limbs during the painful period. Deformity resulted when the healthy muscle in a muscle pair pulled the affected muscle out of shape. Unfortunately, many polio victims treated with immobilization sustained some type of crippling. Elizabeth explained that she successfully treated spasms with moist heat… (Kinney and Ostenso, 1943)

Although many patients who were treated with the Kinney method achieved relief and did not develop deformities, her methods were not endorsed by the medical community in Australia. Instead, she was ridiculed by the medical community and accused of being politically motivated. After the death of her main supporter, Dr. McDonnell, who had stated: "She has knocked our theories into a cocked hat, but her treatment works, and that's all that counts;" she decided to bring her ideas to the United States. (Kinney and Ostenso, 1943)

Following her arrival in America, Kinney again received little support from the medical community. Even though Sister Kinney understood the importance of obtaining medical sanction, she recognized the revolutionary nature of her method… To avoid being labeled a quack Sister Kenny realized that her method had to receive scientific validation (Levine, 1954). Yet, she vacillated between a mission of research and one of instruction. For example, she stated, "I came to America to teach my method—not to enter a research experiment." (Potter, 1941)

Kinney realized that American physicians wanted systematic proof that her empirically demonstrated method worked. But performing a valid experiment on the Kinney method of immobilization raised ethical problems. No parents would allow their children to receive a treatment that was not the most effective that medicine could offer. (Kinney and Ostenso, 1943; Potter, 1941)

1. What is your response to her?

2. What are the major ethical issues involved in the design of this study?

3. How would you design a research study to determine the most effective treatment for spasms in poliomyelitis?

Check your answers with those in Appendix A, Chapter 13.

ACTIVITY 8

Web-Based Activity

Go to the web site www.nursingethics.ca. Take a good look at the URL. From where does this web site originate?

Now click on "Articles." Click on "Professionalism in Nursing: The Struggle to Attain Professional Status." What three things does the author (Moloney) state that nurses still need to do to be recognized as professionals?

POST-TEST

1. A researcher must receive some form of IRB approval (before; after) _____ beginning to conduct research involving humans.

2. If you question whether a researcher has permission to conduct a study in your hospital, you would want to see a document demonstrating approval from which group(s)?

3. Should a researcher list all the possible risks and benefits of participating in a research study? Circle one: Yes   No

4. If you agreed to collect data for a researcher who had not asked the patient's permission to participate in the research study, you would be violating the patient's right to:

The answers to the post-test are in the textbook's web site. Please check with your instructor for these answers.

REFERENCES

Bloom K and Trice L (1997). The efficacy of individualized computerized testing in nursing education, *Computer Nurs* 15:82–88.

Hansen BC and Hansen KD (1995). Academic and scientific misconduct: issues for nursing educators, *J Prof Nurs* 11(1):31–39.

Kang SY, Magura S, and Shapiro JL (1994). Correlates of cocaine/crack use among inner-city incarcerated adolescents, *Am J Drug Alcohol Abuse* 20:413–429.

Oppewal SR (1997). Sister Elizabeth Kinney, an Australian nurse, and treatment of poliomyelitis victims, *Image: J Nurs Schol* 29:83–87.

Rempusheski VE, Wolfe BE, Dow KH, and Fish LC (1996). Peer review by nursing research committees in hospitals, *Image: J Nurs Schol* 28:51–53.

KATHLEEN ROSE-GRIPPA

14

Data Collection Methods

Introduction

> Observe, probe
> Details unfold
> Let nature's secrets
> Be stammeringly retold.
> —Goethe

The focus of this chapter is basic information about data collection. As a consumer of research, the reader needs the skills to evaluate and critique data collection methods in published research studies. In order to achieve these skills it is helpful to have an appreciation of the process or the critical thinking "journey" the researcher has taken to be ready to collect the data. Each of the preceding chapters represented important preliminary steps in the research planning and designing phases prior to data collection. Although most researchers are eager to begin data collection, the planning for data collection is very important. The planning includes identifying and prioritizing data needs, developing or selecting appropriate data collection tools, and selecting and training data collection personnel before proceeding with actual collection of data.

The five types of data collection methods differ in their basic approach and the strengths and weaknesses of their characteristics. Readers should be prepared to ask questions about the appropriateness of the measures chosen by the researcher to gather data about the variable of concern. This includes determining the objectivity, consistency, quantifiability, observer intervention, and/or obtrusiveness of the chosen data collection method.

Learning Outcomes

On completion of this chapter, the reader should be able to do the following:

- Describe the five types of data collection methods used in nursing research.
- Describe the advantages and disadvantages of selected data collection methods.
- Match types of variables to the most appropriate data collection method.
- Critique data collection components of the methodology of specific studies.

- Evaluate the applicability of published research studies based upon a critique of their data collection method.
- Discuss the role of data collection in the overall research process.

ACTIVITY 1

Review each of the articles referenced below; be especially thorough in reading the sections that relate to data collection methods. Answer the questions in relation to what you understand from the article. For some questions, there may be more than one answer.

Study 1

Bull MJ, Hansen HE, and Gross CR (2000). *A professional-patient partnership model of discharge planning with elders hospitalized with heart failure* in Appendix A of the text.

1. Which data collection method(s) is/are used in this research study?
   a. A physiological measure
   b. An observational measure
   c. An interview measure
   d. A questionnaire measure
   e. Records of available data

2. In your opinion what would be the advantage in using this method? What explanation do the investigators provide?

Study 2

Cohen MZ and Ley CD (2000). *Bone marrow transplantation: The battle for hope in the face of fear* in Appendix B of the text.

1. Which data collection method is used in this research study?
   a. A physiological measure
   b. An observational measure
   c. An interview measure
   d. A questionnaire
   e. Records of available data

2. Rationale for appropriateness of data collection method:

3. What is your opinion as to the success of the method chosen?

Study 3

Mahon NE, Yarcheski A, and Yarcheski,TJ (2000). *Positive and negative outcomes of anger in early adolescents* in Appendix C of the textbook.

1. What data collection method is used in this research study?
    a. A physiological measure
    b. An observational measure
    c. An interview measure
    d. A questionnaire
    e. Records of available data

2. What were the strengths in using this method?

Study 4

LoBiondo-Wood G, Williams L, Kouzekanani K, and McGhee C (2000). *Family adaptation to a child's transplant: pretransplant phase* in Appendix D.

1. What data collection method is used in this research study?
    a. A physiological measure
    b. An observational measure
    c. An interview measure
    d. A questionnaire
    e. Records of available data

2. What characteristics of the 29 mothers made the use of this method of data collection reasonable?

Check your answers with those in Appendix A, Chapter 14.

ACTIVITY 2

Using the content of Chapter 14 in the text, have fun with the *Word Search Exercise*. Answer the questions below and find the word in the puzzle.

1. Baccalaureate-prepared nurses are _____ of research.

2. _____ methods are those methods that use technical instruments to collect data about patients' physical, chemical, microbiological, or anatomical status.

3. _____ is the distortion of data as a result of the observer's presence.

4. _____ are best used when it is important to get responses while minimizing bias.

5. _____ as a method of data collection is subject to problems of availability, authenticity, and accuracy.

6. _____ are especially useful when there are finite number of questions to be asked and the questions are clear and specific.

7. Essential in the critique of data collection methods is the emphasis on the appropriateness, _____, and _____ of the method employed.

8. _____ raises ethical questions (especially informed consent issues); therefore, it is not used much in nursing.

9. _____ _____ is the consistency of observations between two or more observers.

10. _____ is the process of translating the concepts/variables into measurable phenomena.

11. _____ is a format that uses closed-ended items, and there are a fixed number of alternative responses.

12. _____ is the method for objective, systematic, and quantitative description of communications and documentary evidence.

13. This exercise is supposed to be _____!

```
N Z B Z G P M X N G L A C I G O L O I S Y H P W G
P C Z C J N Z Y I H N H G Z M B T E C B C I Y W D
M N R E A C T I V I T Y O Y Y D X E X Q U P O J T
E Q A I V U C W P C L B F F H V H I X G V T Z I X
B I D V L E T N E M L A E C N O C N L S N Z N O D
W H V F Y Q J V G A M C N Y X O O V O T P P R P Y
U E D G G W D V G L A P T V N T A Y Q F U N F E T
G G X R G P B E E E X O Z S B I X Y F A Y X O R I
W S C R N D H X U Z Y P U M H A Z M D G N D R A V
S V C F M B R F Y X C M I B E E O B P K S G U T I
T Y T I L I B A I L E R R E T A R R E T N I Q I T
U N L V D Y H R H R S E N L Y L H B F F W J U O C
S V L B O H Y S S W F J H L O G V H R N S C E N E
T X L K C O N T E N T A N A L Y S I S V Y K S A J
C O N S I S T E N C Y R O R Q I S M A K R R T L B
O Y X G J N Z L I K E R T S C A L E K E C Q I I O
M N Q V Z R J S W E I V R E T N I A E Z C D O Z E
A J Z Z Y H H E N O W T R E F O W Q U H N I N A Y
E S K K D D G Z T J L R T T C D T O Z E N G N T T
P Z X Z P B F T C U A P B H K O Z O P T R J A I K
N Q Q D V B L O P L F B V B C O R X C Q C X I O J
G V X B B W K L B R U P G H Z B B D P I R Y R N W
Y U G Y F M D A L O F O X D Y P Y E S P J H E N U
S I C N M A O J F M K T N Y Y V Z S I P E D S M T
W Q T U D R W I B Y R G C C A S L C G O R P B U Y
```

Check your answers with those in Appendix A, Chapter 14.

ACTIVITY 3

You are reviewing a study and concealment is necessary. In other words, there is no other way to collect the data and the data collected will not have negative consequences for the subject.

1. Name at least one population where concealment is not uncommon.

2.   How would you obtain subjects' consent?

3.   What is the major reason for using concealment?

Check your answers with those in Appendix A, Chapter 14.

ACTIVITY 4

You are asked to participate in discussions about impending research in your community. The purpose of the study is to identify the health status, beliefs, practices, preventive services currently known and used and accessibility/availability of health service needs for the residents of your rural community.

Take me on your critical thinking journey…

Describe what you would consider in the selection of a data collection method. Review each method and discuss the pros and cons for choosing a specific data collection method. State your rationale for your final selection. What would be your thinking about instruments and types?

Check your answers with those in Appendix A, Chapter 14.

ACTIVITY 5

Using the content of Chapter 14 in the textbook, circle the correct response for each question. Some questions will have more than one answer.

1. What is a primary advantage of physiological measures?
   a. The measuring tool never affects the phenomena that are being measured
   b. One of the easiest types of methods to implement
   c. The unlikelihood that study participants/subjects can distort the physiological information
   d. Their objectivity, sensitivity, and precision
   e. All of the above

2. Self-report measures are usually more useful than observation measures in obtaining information about which of the following?
   a. Socially unacceptable or private behaviors
   b. Complex research situations when it is difficult to separate processes and interactions
   c. When the researcher is interested in character traits
   d. All of the above

3. Which of the following would be considered disadvantages of using observational data collection methods?
   a. Individual bias may interfere with the data collection.
   b. Ethical concerns may be increasingly significant to researchers using observational data collection methods.
   c. Individual judgments and values influence the perceptions of the observers.
   d. All of the above.

4. In nursing research, when might questionnaires be used as an appropriate method for data collection?
   a. Whenever expense is a concern for the researcher
   b. When a researcher is interested in obtaining information directly from the subjects
   c. When the researcher needs to collect data from a large group of subjects who are not easily accessible
   d. When accuracy is of the utmost importance to the researcher

5. Which of the following would be considered advantages of using existing records or available data to answer a research question?
   a. The use of available data reduces the risk of researcher bias in data collection.
   b. Time involvement in the research study can be reduced by the use of available records or data.
   c. Consistent collection of information over periods of time allows the researcher to study trends.
   d. All of the above.

Check your answers with those in Appendix A, Chapter 14.

ACTIVITY 6

Web-Based Activity

Go to www.mriresearch.org—the current project of Midwest Research Institute (MRI) is the development of the NDNQI.

1. What do these initials mean?

2. How many quality indicators form the core of NDNQI?

Scroll down to "Sample Data Collection Instruments." Click on it and then click on the "Monthly Patient Fall Report." Into what category of data collection instruments would you place this form?

Check your answers with those in Appendix A, Chapter 14.

POST-TEST

Read each question thoroughly and then circle the correct answer. For some questions more than one answer may be correct.

1. What is the process of translating concepts that are of interest to the researcher into observable and measurable phenomena?
   a. Objectivism
   b. Systematization
   c. Subjectivism
   d. Operationalization

2. Answering research questions pertaining to psychosocial variables can best be answered by using which data gathering technique(s)?
   a. Observation
   b. Interviews
   c. Questionnaires
   d. All of the above

3. What is collection of data from each subject in the same or in a similar manner known as?
   a. Repetition
   b. Dualism
   c. Consistency
   d. Recidivism

4. What is consistency of observations between two or more observers known as?
   a. Intrarater reliability
   b. Interrater reliability
   c. Consistency reliability
   d. Repetitive reliability

5. Physiological and biological measurement might be used by nurse researchers when studying which of these variables?
   a. A comparison of student nurses' ACT scores and their GPAs
   b. Hypertensive clients' responses to a stress test
   c. Children's dietary patterns
   d. The degree of pain relief achieved following guided imagery

6. Scientific observations should fulfill which of the following conditions?
   a. Observations are consistent with the study objectives
   b. Observations are standardized and systematically recorded
   c. Observations are checked and controlled
   d. All of the above

7. In a research study, a participant observer spent regularly scheduled hours in a homeless shelter and occasionally stayed overnight. The people staying in the home were told that this person was conducting a research study. The researcher freely engaged in conversation and openly observed the homeless. What is the observational role of the researcher?
   a. Concealment without intervention
   b. Concealment with intervention
   c. No concealment without intervention
   d. No concealment with intervention

8. In unstructured observation, which of the following might occur?
   a. Extensive field notes are recorded
   b. Subjects are informed what behaviors are being observed
   c. The researcher frequently records interesting anecdotes
   d. All of the above

9. Which of the following is not consistent with a Likert scale?
   a. It contains closed-ended items.
   b. It contains open-ended items.
   c. It contains lists of statements.
   d. Items are evaluated on the amount of agreement.

10. Although it is acceptable to use multiple instruments within a research study, the study is more acceptable if only one method is used for the data collection.
    a. True
    b. False

11. Social desirability is seldom a concern for researchers when the data collection method used in the study is interviews.
    a. True
    b. False

12. A researcher desires to use a questionnaire in a study but cannot find one that will gather the information desired about a particular variable. The decision is made to develop a new instrument. Which of the following should the researcher do?
    a. Define the construct, formulate the items, and assess the items for content validity
    b. Develop instructions for users and pilot the instrument
    c. Estimate reliability and validity
    d. All of the above

13. The researcher who invests significant amounts of time in the development of an instrument has a professional responsibility to publish the results.
    a. True
    b. False

14. In order to evaluate the adequacy of various data collection methods, which of the following should be observed in the written research report?
    a. Clear identification of the rationale for selecting a physiological measure
    b. The problems of bias and reactivity are addressed with observational measures
    c. There is a clear explanation of how interviews were conducted and how interviewers were trained
    d. All of the above

15. In conducting a research study, the researcher has a responsibility to ensure that all study subjects received the same information and data was collected from all participants in the same manner.
    a. True
    b. False

The answers to the post-test are in the textbook's web site. Please check with your instructor for these answers.

REFERENCES

Bull MJ, Hansen HE, and Gross CR (2000). A professional-patient partnership model of discharge planning with elders hospitalized with heart failure, *Appl Nurs Res* 13(1):19–28.

Cohen MZ and Ley CD (2000). Bone marrow transplantation: the battle for hope in the face of fear, *Oncol Nurs Forum* 27(3):473–480.

LoBiondo-Wood G, Williams L, Kouzekanani K, and McGhee C (2000). Family adaptation to a child's transplant: pretransplant phase, *Progress in Transplantation* 10(2):81–87.

Mahon NE, Yarcheski A, and Yarcheski T (2000). Positive and negative outcomes of anger in early adolescents, *Res Nurs Health* 23:17–24.

KATHLEEN ROSE-GRIPPA

15

Reliability and Validity

Introduction

If someone tells you, "Hey, I found a new restaurant that you will really love," you will consider that information from at least two perspectives before you spend your money there. First, does this person know what she is talking about when it comes to your taste in food? Second, has this person given you good information about food in the past?

You answer "no" to the first question. You prefer seafood served in an elegant setting, and your friend prefers pizza served in a place with sawdust on the floor. Using this information you will consider her opinion to be invalid for you. You will never give this restaurant another thought.

But if you answer "yes" to the first question because you share similar tastes in food, you will move on to the second question. You remember the tough fettuccini, the superb Southern fried chicken, the unbaked pizza dough and the hockey puck biscuits from earlier recommendations. It is likely that while you and your friend share food preferences, her information is not reliable. You can't trust her to give you good information over time. If you are feeling like an adventure, you may try the new restaurant or you may not.

Validity and reliability of the data collection instruments used in a study are to be regarded in the same way that you would consider your friend's advice about restaurants. Is the instrument valid? Does it provide accurate information? Is the instrument reliable? Does it provide consistent information whenever it is used? Consideration of both validity and reliability influences your confidence in the results of the study.

Learning Outcomes

On completion of this chapter, the student should be able to do the following:

- Discuss reliability and validity as they relate to data collection instruments.
- Compare content, criterion, and construct validity in the choice of instruments used in research.
- Compare stability, homogeneity, and equivalence in determining reliability.
- Critique the reliability and validity reported in research studies.

ACTIVITY 1

Either random error (R) or systematic error (S) may occur in a research study. For each of the following examples, identify the type of measurement error and how the error might be corrected.

1. _____ The scale used to obtain daily weights was inaccurate by 3 pounds less than actual weight.
   Correction:

2. _____ Students chose the socially acceptable responses on an instrument to assess attitudes toward AIDS patients.
   Correction:

3. _____ Confusion existed among the evaluators on how to score the wound healing.
   Correction:

4. _____ The subjects were nervous about taking the psychological tests.
   Correction:

Check your answers with those in Appendix A, Chapter 15.

ACTIVITY 2

Validity is the concern whether the measurement tools are actually measuring what they are supposed to measure. Use the terms from the following list to complete each of the items in this activity.

Concurrent validity   Content validity   Contrasted groups
Construct validity   Convergent validity   Criterion-related validity
Divergent validity   Face validity   Factor analysis
Multitrait-multimethod approach   Hypothesis testing   Predictive validity
Rating from a panel of experts

1. ". . . the 105 items, an obstetric history form, and demographic questions were mailed to a convenience sample of 446 women with and without children who had experienced at least one miscarriage within the previous 10 years. Through this study the 105 items were reduced to 30 psychometrically sound items. _____ was established by examining the capacity of the Impact of Miscarriage Scale to discriminate among groups of women for whom miscarriage would be expected to hold different meanings. Significant differences. . . were found for women with and without children, with and without a history of late-gestation pregnancy losses, and with fewer than three versus three or more miscarriages. . ." (Swanson, 1999)

2.   _____ is an intuitive, preliminary type of instrument evaluation.

3.   "A written 31-item multiple choice survey was developed to obtain information on nurses' attitudes and perceived barriers to pain management with opioids when caring for patients with sickle cell pain episodes. The survey was divided into three components. . . The survey was favorably reviewed by the Nursing Research Committee (composed of advanced practice nurses, unit managers, and staff nurses) for _____ before distribution." (Pack-Mabien, Labbe, Herbert, and Haynes, 2001)

4.   The study addressed the effects of spiritual activities on adaptational outcomes, e.g. emotional distress and quality of life, in women with HIV. " The scales used in the analysis were initially constructed using standardized procedures. Validity of the scales was evaluated using exploratory factor analyses. Initial results supported the _____ of the scales, with items for each scale loading on a common factor (factor loadings .400 or higher)." (Sowell, Moneyham, Hennessy, Guillor, Demi, and Seals, 2000)

5.   "Previous studies have demonstrated that the Daily Hassles for Adolescents Inventory has good _____, as evidenced by its significant relationship to adjustment measures." (Guthrie, Young, Williams, Boyd, and Kintner, 2002)

6.   Construct validity, an assessment of the relationship between the instrument and the underlying theory, can be measured in several ways. List three of these: _____, _____, and _____.

7.   "Previous reports have provided evidence of the instrument's reliability and validity: internal consistency for the total scale was .88, and correlations with various cognitive measures were as high as .72." (Badr, 2001) This is an example of _____ validity which is one way of measuring _____ validity.

Check your answers with those in Appendix A, Chapter 15.

ACTIVITY 3

An instrument is considered reliable if it is accurate and consistent. If the concept being studied is stable, the same results should occur when measurement is repeated.

1.   Three concepts related to reliability include _____, _____, and _____.

2.   Give an example of each of the two types of tests for stability.

3. In what instance would it be better to use an alternate form rather than a test-retest measure for stability?

4. Homogeneity is a measure of internal consistency. All items on the instrument should be complementary and measure the same characteristic or concepts. For each of the following examples, identify which of the following tests for homogeneity is described:
    (1) Item-total correlations
    (2) Split-half reliability
    (3) Kuder-Richardson (KR-20) coefficient
    (4) Cronbach's alpha

    a. _____ The odd items of the test had a high correlation with the even numbers of the test.

    b. _____ Each item on the test using a 5-point Likert scale had a moderate correlation with every other item on the test.

    c. _____ Each item on the test ranged in correlation from 0.62 to 0.89 with the total.

    d. _____ Each item on the true-false test had a moderate correlation with every other item on the test.

5. a. Review Table 2 in the Bull, Hansen, and Gross (2000) study found in Appendix A of the textbook. Think about the concept of face validity. Think about the variables being addressed in the study. Would you conclude that these instruments had face validity for this study?

    b. What information is given to the reader in Columns 4 and 5 of Table 2?

    c. How does this information influence your level of confidence in the results of this study?

Check your answers with those in Appendix A, Chapter 15.

ACTIVITY 4

Web-Based Activity

Go to www.cdc.gov. Click on "Health Topics A-Z," then on "H," then on "Health-Related Quality of Life," and then on "Methods and Measures." Scroll to "Measurement Properties" and click. Scroll to the Nelson, Holtzman, Bolen, Stanwyck, and Mack article and click on it. Read the first part of the article. What measures of health-related quality of life are considered to have high reliability and high validity?

ACTIVITY 5

In this activity you will use the critiquing criteria listed in Chapter 15 (p. 327) of the textbook to think about the Mahon, Yarcheski, and Yarcheski (2000) study in Appendix C of the textbook.

1.   How many instruments for data collection were used in this study?

2.   Read the validity and reliability information provided for each instrument and answer the critiquing questions in Chapter 15. Complete the table below using "Y" for yes and "N" for no.

Critiquing Questions

Instrument	#1	#2	#3	#4	#5	#6	#7
State Anger							
Trait Anger							
AGWB							
Symptom Pattern							
Vigor-Activity							
Change Subscale							

POST-TEST

Using the following terms, complete the sentences for the type of validity or reliability discussed. Terms may be used more than once.

Content validity   Test-retest reliability   Divergent validity
Factor analysis   Cronbach's alpha   Interrater reliability
Convergent validity   Alternate or parallel form   Concurrent validity

1. In tests for reliability the self-efficacy scale had a(n) _____ of 0.88, demonstrating internal consistency for the new measure.

2. The ABC social support scale demonstrated _____ with correlation of 0.84 with the XYZ interpersonal relationships scale.

3. _____ was supported with a correlation of 0.42 between the ABC social support scale and the QRS loneliness scale.

4. The investigator established _____ through evaluation of the cardiac recovery scale by a panel of cardiac clinical nurse specialists. All items were rated 0 to 5 for importance to recovery and only items scoring above an average of 3 were kept in the final scale.

5. The results of the _____ were that all the items clustered around three factors, lending support to the notion that there are three dimensions of coping.

6. The observations were rated by three experts. The _____ among the observers was 94%.

7. To assess _____, subjects completed the locus of control questionnaire at the beginning of the project and 2 weeks later. The correlation of 0.86 supports the stability of the concept.

8. Bennett et al. (1996) developed an instrument: the Cardiac Event Threat Questionnaire (CTQ). They established _____ by reviewing the literature, reviewing concerns identified by patients recovering from a cardiac event, and had the items critiqued by a panel of experts.

9. The results of the CTQ that measured threat were highly correlated with the results of a test measuring negative emotions. This established _____.

10. Bennett et al. (1996) reported that internal consistency reliabilities of the five factors of the CTQ were computed with the _____ statistic.

The answers to the post-test are in the textbook's web site. Please check with your instructor for these answers.

REFERENCES

Badr (Zahr) LK (2001). Quantitative and qualitative predictors of development for low-birth-weight infants of Latino background, *Appl Nurs Res* 14(4):125–135.

Bennett SJ et al. (1996): Development of an instrument to measure threat related to cardiac events, *Nurs Res* 45:266–270.

Bull MJ, Hansen HE, and Gross CR (2000). A professional-patient partnership model of discharge planning with elders hospitalized with heart failure, *Appl Nurs Res* 13(1):19–28.

Flynn L (1997). The health practices of homeless women: a causal model, *Nurs Res* 46:72–77.

Guthrie BJ, Young AM, Williams DR, Boyd CJ, and Kintner, EK (2002). African-American girls' smoking habits and day-to-day experience with racial discrimination, *Nurs Res* 51(3):183–190.

Mahon NE, Yarcheski A, and Yarcheski TJ (2000). Positive and negative outcomes of anger in early adolescents, *Res in Nurs Hlth* 23:17–24.

Pack-Mabien A, Labbe E, Herbert D, and Haynes J Jr (2001). Nurses' attitudes and practices in sickle cell pain management, *Appl Nurs Res* 14(4):187–192.

Sowell R, Moneyham L, Hennessy M, Guillory J, Demi A, and Seals B (2000). Spiritual activities as a resistance resource for women with human immunodeficiency virus, *Nurs Res* 49(2):73–82.

Swanson KM (1999). Research-based practice with women who have had miscarriages, *Image: Journal of Nursing Scholarship* 31(4):339–345.

KATHLEEN ROSE-GRIPPA

16

Descriptive Data Analysis

Introduction

Measurement is critical to any study. The researcher begins to think about how to measure the variables while reading the literature and thinking through the theoretical rationale for the study. Formulating the operational definitions is often the first direct link to the concept of measurement. These operational definitions point to relevant data collection instruments that in turn point to data analysis strategies. Seldom does a researcher have the luxury of defining the variables exactly as desired leading to ideal data collection instrument(s) that perfectly match analytical strategies. Your task as a critical reader of research is to consider all of the steps taken by the researcher and then ask "Did the researcher use the descriptive statistical tools that provide the clearest possible summary of the data?"

Some studies will rely on descriptive statistics as the major data analysis strategy, and other studies will use a combination of descriptive and inferential statistics. The majority of studies will utilize descriptive statistics to provide readers with general information about the sample; e.g., the gender, age, and level of education of those who participated in the study. The choice of descriptive or inferential statistics to answer the question posed by the researcher will vary as the complexity of the research question and the information needs of the audience vary.

The focus of this chapter is on the use of descriptive statistics. First, the exercises in this chapter will provide you with some practice in working with the concept of measurement. Second, you will have the opportunity to think through some of the decisions relevant to the use of descriptive statistics.

Learning Objectives

On completion of this chapter, the student should be able to do the following:

- Distinguish among the four levels of measurement.
- Identify the level of measurement used in specified sets of data.
- Recognize the symbols associated with specific descriptive statistical tools.
- Interpret accurate measures of central tendency and measures of variation.
- Critically evaluate the use of descriptive statistics in specified studies.

ACTIVITY 1

Match the level of measurement found in Column B with the appropriate example(s) in Column A. The levels of measurement in Column B will be used more than once.

	Column A		**Column B**
1. _____	Amount of emesis	a.	Nominal
2. _____	Scores on the ACT, SAT, or the GRE	b.	Ordinal
3. _____	Height or weight	c.	Interval
4. _____	High, moderate, or low level of social support	d.	Ratio
5. _____	Satisfaction with nursing care		
6. _____	Use or nonuse of contraception		
7. _____	Amount of empathy		
8. _____	Number of feet or meters walked		
9. _____	Type A or Type B behavior		
10. _____	Body temperature measured with centigrade thermometer		

Check your answers with those in Appendix A, Chapter 16.

ACTIVITY 2

Read the following excerpts from specific studies. Identify both the independent and dependent variable(s) and indicate what level of measurement would apply. You may find the Critical Thinking Decision Path from Chapter 16 (page 333) of the textbook to be very helpful in answering these questions.

1. "The visual analog scale (VAS) was chosen because it is used frequently in pain management. In addition, Price, McGrath, Rafii, and Buckingham (1983) have previously established it as a reliable and valid pain measurement instrument. This tool is well-known within the literature and in clinical practice." (Hattula, McGovern, and Neumann, 2002)

   Note: The VAS is a 10-centimeter line with the words "no pain" at one end of the line and the words "worst possible pain" at the other end of the line. Clients indicate their current pain experience by marking the line at the point that best describes their pain.

   a.   Name the variable of interest.

   b.   Identify the level of measurement of this variable.

2.   "This study examined differences between blacks and whites in delay times and types of clinical symptoms of MI, and the effect of differences in race and types of clinical symptoms on prehospital delay time." (Lee, Bahler, Chung, Alonzo, and Zeller, 2000)

   a.   Name the independent variable(s).

   b.   Name the dependent variable(s).

   c.   Identify the level of measurement of each variable.

3.   This study examined the effectiveness of a psychoeducational intervention delivered over 12 weeks… Experimental and control groups did not differ in emotional health, functional health status, or satisfaction."

Emotional health was measured with an instrument that asks subjects to report the frequency of experience with a list of 16 symptoms of depression within the past week. *Functional health status* was measured using a standardized, 10-item pictorial self-report instrument. Subject rates self on a 5-point scale with higher values indicating poorer functioning.
Satisfaction was measured with a 21-item scale. Subjects rated nurses on skill in caring for clients, teaching, and providing information. (Lenz and Perkins, 2000)

   a.   Name the independent variable(s).

   b.   Name the dependent variable(s).

   c.   Identify the level of measurement of each variable.

4.   "The physiological indicators of anxiety, including HR [heart rate], SBP [systolic blood pressure], and DBP [diastolic blood pressure], were measured on admission to the endoscopy unit, 5 minutes after receiving a standard preprocedure medication, 5 minutes after the procedure, and immediately before discharge from the endoscopy unit." (Smolen, Topp, and Singer, 2002)

   a.   Name the variable(s).

   b.   Identify the level of measurement of each variable.

Check your answers with those in Appendix A, Chapter 16.

ACTIVITY 3

1. In Activity 2 you identified the level of measurement for several variables. You now need to use this information to think about some the analytical treatment of data. This activity includes the report of data from two of the studies used in Activity 2. Your task is to look at the report of the data, think about the level of measurement information, and decide if the appropriate descriptive statistic was used. Again, you may find the Critical Thinking Decision Path from Chapter 16 of the textbook useful.

Table 4. Prevalence of Typical and Atypical Clinical Symptoms of Myocardial Infarction

Symptom	Total (%) (N = 128)	Black (%) (N = 41)	White (%) (N = 87)
Chest pain	77.1	78.0	76.5
Pain in shoulder, neck, and jaw	38.9	29.3	43.5
Dyspnea*	32.8	56.1	23.5
Perspiration	32.1	41.5	29.4
Nausea/vomiting	28.2	24.4	30.6
Fatigue*	21.4	31.7	16.5
Palpitation	6.1	9.8	4.7
No symptoms	3.8	0.0	5.9

*$p<.05$.

Lee H, Bahler R, Chung C, Alonzo A, and Zeller, RA (2000). Prehospital delay with myocardial infarction: The interactive effect of clinical symptoms and race, *Appl Nurs Res* 13(3):129.

a. Review your answer from item b in Activity 2 of this chapter. What is the variable of interest in this table?

b. Name the types of statistics used to describe the information.

c. Using the Critical Thinking Decision Path found in Chapter 16 of the textbook, what level of measurement is needed to use the statistic you identified?

d. Does the level of measurement named in your answer to the previous question match the level of measurement you identified in item b of Activity 2?
Yes   No

e. Did the investigators use an appropriate statistic in this table?
Yes   No

2. The next table is from the Smolen, Topp, and Singer (2002) study used in item d of
    Activity 2.

Table 2. Differences in Sedation Requirements and Duration of Procedure

Variables	Dosage	SD	df	t	p
Versed (mg)					
Music	2.13	0.72	30	4.9	.000[a]
Nonmusic	3.81	1.17			
Demerol (mg)					
Music	64.38	23.57	30	3.9	.000[a]
Nonmusic	96.56	23.01			
Procedure time (min)					
Music	26.63	12.43	30	1.6	.125
Nonmusic	32.88	9.79			

[a]$p<.05$.

Smolen D, Topp R, and Singer L (2002). The effect of self-selected music during colonoscopy on
anxiety, heart rate, and blood pressure, *Appl Nurs Res*, 16(2):130.

a. Identify the variables represented in Table 2.

b. Which level of measurement would fit each of these variables?

c. Table 2 contains both descriptive and inferential (Chapter 17) statistics. Is this
    appropriate given the level of measurement of the data?
    Yes   No

d. Which columns of Table 2 contain descriptive data?

e. What information does the "standard deviation" give you?

ACTIVITY 4

If you have taken a course in statistics, you are familiar with the statistical notation used to refer to specific types of descriptive statistics. This activity will serve as a quick review. For those of you who have not yet taken a statistics course, this exercise will provide enough information for you to recognize some of the statistical notations.

This is a *reverse* crossword puzzle; therefore, the puzzle is already completed. Your task is to identify the appropriate clue for each answer found in the puzzle. List the correct answers in the spaces provided on the next page.

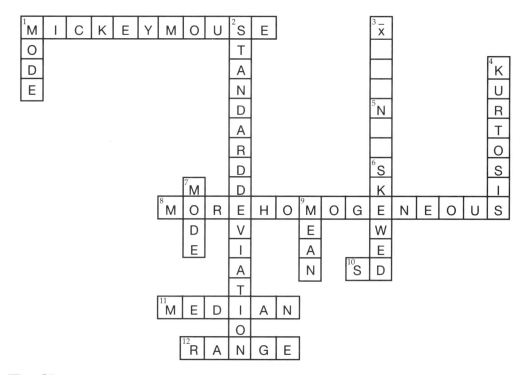

The Clues

a. Measure of central tendency used with interval or ratio data
b. Abbreviation for the number of measures in a given data set (the measures may be individual people or some smaller piece of data like blood pressure readings)
c. Measure of variation that shows the lowest and highest number in a data set
d. Can describe the height of a distribution
e. Old abbreviation for the mean
f. Marks the "score" where 50% of the scores are higher and 50% are lower
g. Describes a distribution characterized by a tail
h. Abbreviation for standard deviation
i. 68% of the values in a normal distribution fall between ±1 of this statistic
j. Goofy's best friend
k. Very unstable

l. The values that occur most frequently in a data set.

m. Describes a set of data with a standard deviation of 3 when compared to a set of data with a standard deviation of 12.

Across

1.

3.

5.

8.

10.

11.

12.

Down

1.

2.

4.

6.

7.

9.

ACTIVITY 5

You have now had some experience with matching variables, levels of measurement, and types of descriptive statistics. It is time to move to the interpretation and critiquing of the use of descriptive statistics. Table 4 from a study conducted by Jordan, Price, and Fitzgerald (2000) follows. Study the information in Table 4 below and answer the questions that follow.

Table 4. Parental Support for Sexuality Education in Various Settings/Various Age Groups

Rural Setting	Elementary Grade*		Junior High		High School	
	N	(%)	N	(%)	N	(%)
School	255	(68)	342	(91)	341	(91)
Doctor's office	211	(56)	294	(79)	312	(83)
Health department	215	(57)	292	(77)	311	(83)
Church	160	(43)	255	(68)	270	(72)

N = 374

*Parents could select more than one response per grade level.

Jordan TR, Price JH, and Fitzgerald S (2000). Rural parents' communication with their teenagers about sexual issues, *Journal of School Health* 70(8):338–344. Reprinted with permission. American School Health Association, Kent, Ohio.

1. What is/are the highest percentage(s) reported?

2. With which groups are these percentages associated?

3. For which age group was the range of scores the greatest?

4. The following text is the investigators' discussion of the data in Table 4. Does the information in the table and the text agree?

To determine parental preferences regarding when sexuality education should begin, and in what venues it should be taught, parents were asked to indicate whether they favored sexuality education for three different age groups (elementary, junior high, and high school) in four different rural settings (school, church, doctor's office, health department). Overall, parents supported offering sexuality education in most venues for all age groups (Table 4). For all age groups of students, parents most consistently supported the school as their favored venue of the four (68% to 91%). Support for sexuality education at each venue increased with the age of the proposed target audience. Of the four choices, the church was the least-supported educational venue for sexuality education (48% to 78%). (Jordan, Price, and Fitzgerald, p. 342)

Check your answers with those in Appendix A, Chapter 16

ACTIVITY 6

Using the studies in Appendices A-D in the textbook, answer the following questions regarding the use of descriptive statistics in each study. Once again, use the Critical Thinking Decision Path in Chapter 16 of the textbook.

1. Based on the questions asked, was the use of descriptive statistics appropriate for this study?

   a. Bull, Hansen, and Gross

   b. Cohen and Ley

   c. Mahon, Yarcheski, and Yarcheski

   d. LoBiondo-Wood, Williams, Kouzekanani, and McGhee

2. Were descriptive statistics used in the study?

   a. Bull, Hansen, and Gross

   b. Cohen and Ley

   c. Mahon, Yarcheski, and Yarcheski

   d. LoBiondo-Wood, Williams, Kouzekanani, and McGhee

3. What data were summarized and/or explained through the use of descriptive statistics?

    a. Bull, Hansen, and Gross

    b. Cohen and Ley

    c. Mahon, Yarcheski, and Yarcheski

    d. LoBiondo-Wood, Williams, Kouzekanani, and McGhee

4. Were the descriptive statistics used appropriately?

    a. Bull, Hansen, and Gross

    b. Cohen and Ley

    c. Mahon, Yarcheski, and Yarcheski

    d. LoBiondo-Wood, Williams, Kouzekanani, and McGhee

5. Which of the four studies relied the most heavily on the use of descriptive statistics?

Check your answers in Appendix A, Chapter 1

ACTIVITY 7

Web-Based Activity

Go to www.yahooligans.com and click on "Animals" and then "Mammals." Scroll to the "Carnivores" section of the index. Click on "Northern River Otter." What descriptive statistics are provided on the Northern River Otter?

POST-TEST

1. Two outpatient clinics measured client waiting time as one indicator of effectiveness. The mean and standard deviation of waiting time in minutes is reported below. Which outpatient clinic would you prefer, assuming that all other things are equal? Explain your answer.

	Clinic 1	**Clinic 2**
Mean (in minutes)	40	25
Standard deviation (in minutes)	10	45

2. You are responsible for ordering a new supply of hospital gowns for your unit. Which measure of central tendency would be the most useful in your decision making? Explain your answer.

3. Use Table 5 that follows and answer the following questions.

   a. How many total subjects participated in this study?

   b. What advice would men most frequently give to someone newly diagnosed with human papillomavirus infection (HPV)?

   c. Do the men and women agree about the advice they would be the most likely to give to someone newly diagnosed with HPV? Explain your answer.

Table 5. Types of Helpful Advice and Information

	n(%) Respondents	n(%) Women	n(%) Men
Balanced Perspective			
Maintain a positive outlook	39 (44)	27 (44)	12 (44)
Remember you are not alone	20 (23)	15 (25)	5 (19)
Avoid self-blame and negative self-evaluation	18 (21)	17 (28)	1 (4)
Remember that time will heal	8 (9)	8 (13)	0 (0)
Treatment			
Seek treatment for yourself	44 (50)	30 (49)	14 (52)
Realize that warts are treatable	9 (10)	6 (10)	3 (11)
Establish a positive relationship with health care provider	8 (9)	7 (11)	1 (4)
Be realistic about future course of disease	5 (6)	3 (5)	2 (7)
Check yourself for recurrences	3 (3)	2 (3)	1 (4)
Seek evaluation for partners	2 (2)	2 (3)	0 (0)
Sexual Behavior			
Practice safer sex	34 (39)	20 (33)	14 (52)
Inform sexual partners	14 (16)	11 (18)	3 (11)
Knowledge			
Educate yourself and ask questions	21 (24)	15 (25)	6 (22)
Expect inconsistent information	4 (5)	3 (5)	1 (4)
Self Care			
Seek emotional support	11 (13)	11 (18)	0 (0)
Maintain a healthy lifestyle	11 (13)	7 (11)	4 (15)
Other			
Not codable	8 (9)	6 (10)	2 (7)
Having genital warts did not affect me in any way	3 (3)	3 (5)	0 (0)
I don't know what to tell others	1 (1)	0 (0)	1 (4)

Taylor CA, Keller ML, Egan JJ (1997). Advice from affected persons about living with human papillomavirus infection, *Image: J Nurs Schol* 29(1):27–32.

Answers to the post-test items are on the textbook's web site. Check with your instructor for these answers.

REFERENCES

Bull MJ, Hansen HE, and Gross CR (2000). A professional-patient partnership model of discharge planning with elders hospitalized with heart failure, *Appl Nurs Res* 13(1):19–28.

Cohen MZ and Ley CD (2000). Bone marrow transplantation: The battle for hope in the face of fear, *Oncol Nurs Forum* 27(3):473–480.

Hattula JL, McGovern EK, and Neumann TL (2002). Comparison of intravenous cannulation injectable preanesthetics in an adult medical inpatient population, *Appl Nurs Res,* 16(3):189–193.

Jordan TR, Price JH, and Fitzgerald S (2000). Rural parents' communication with their teenagers about sexual issues, *Journal of School Health,* 70(8):338–344.

Lee H, Bahler R, Chung C, Alonzo A, and Zeller RA (2000). Prehospital delay with myocardial infarction: The interactive effect of clinical symptoms and race, *Appl Nurs Res,* 13(3):125–133.

Lenz ER and Perkins S (2000). Coronary artery bypass graft surgery patients and their family member caregivers: Outcomes of a family-focused staged psychoeducational intervention, *Appl Nurs Res* 13(3):142–150

LoBiondo-Wood G, Williams L, Kouzekanani K, and McGhee C (2000). Family adaptation to a child's transplant: Pretransplant phase, *Progress in Transplantation* 10(2):81–87.

Mahon NE, Yarcheski A, and Yarcheski TJ (2000). Positive and negative outcomes of anger in early adolescents, *Res in Nurs and Hlth* 23:17–24.

Smolen D, Topp R, and Singer L (2002). The effect of self-selected music during colonoscopy on anxiety, heart rate, and blood pressure, *Appl Nurs Res* 16(2):126–136.

Taylor CA, Keller ML, Egan JJ (1997). Advice from affected persons about living with human papillomavirus infection, *Image: J Nurs Schol* 29(1):27–32.

KATHLEEN ROSE-GRIPPA

17

Inferential Data Analysis

Introduction

Descriptive statistics are valuable for summarizing data and allowing us to look at salient features about a group of data, but practitioners usually want more information. They want to be able to read about an intervention used with a specific group of individuals and consider the usefulness of that intervention with the clients in their care. These decisions require practitioners to be comfortable with the assumption that the clients in the study and the clients in their care are members of the same population and that the clinical outcomes are a result of the intervention. The researcher's use of inferential statistics in the data analysis is one strategy for building confidence in that critical assumption.

Initially, the numbers, symbols, and tables used to present inferential statistics are intimidating. You can take several steps to reduce that intimidation factor: Take a deep breath and jump in. Remember you have the intelligence and the skills to do this. Learn to look at the array of numbers and symbols one step at a time. Continue to read clinically relevant research. This chapter is designed to help you with the skills part of the task. We will spend a bit of time reviewing the logic underlying inferential statistics, take a look at some specific inferential tools, and spend the bulk of our effort digesting data from the studies included in the text.

Learning Outcomes

On completion of this chapter, the student should be able to do the following:

- Identify the symbols representing specified inferential statistical techniques.
- Choose an appropriate inferential statistical strategy for specified research hypotheses.
- Interpret the results of specified inferential statistical tests.
- Critique the use of inferential statistics in given studies.

ACTIVITY 1

Shortcuts are wonderful. Memorizing the statistical notation saves a lot of time that would be spent flipping through pages looking for the symbol.

The following lists the inferential statistical tools as they appear in Tables 17-1 and 17-2 in the textbook (before beginning this activity, read through the list):

Technique	Notation
Pearson product moment correlation	r
Phi coefficient	ϕ
Kendall's tau	τ
Spearman rho	rs
Multiple analysis of variance (MANOVA)	F
Multiple regression	R
Path analysis	None used
Canonical correlation	Rc
Contingency coefficient	None used
Discriminant function analysis	None used
Logistic regression	None used
t-statistic	t
ANOVA	F
Chi-square	χ^2
Signed rank	Z
Mann Whitney U	U
Analysis of covariance (ANCOVA)	F

Now, obtain the following supplies: a package of 3 x 5 index cards, preferably lined on one side; six pens or a combination of pens and highlighters that will give you six different colors; one broad-tipped, black-ink marker.

You are to create your own set of "statistical assistants." Once they are finished carry them with you when you go to the library. Use them when you are reading reports of research. Before long you will be able to read a piece of research without referring to your stack of statistical assistants.

Once this activity is completed, you will have a set of quick reference cards and a set of flash cards that can be used for memorization exercises.

1. Make your key card first. Take one of the cards and on the side without lines, using the broad-tipped, black marker write *NAME OF INFERENTIAL STATISTICAL TECHNIQUE*.

2. Turn the card over and use the side with lines. Choose one of the pens with colored ink and on the first line, write *Symbol*. Complete this side of the card with five more categories of information using a different line and a different color of ink for each line for each category. The lined side of the card should look like this:

Symbol
# of independent variables (IV)   # of dependent variables (DV)
IV's level of measurement
DV's level of measurement
HR = relationship? (# of variables?)   differences? (# of groups?)
Parametric/nonparametric

Of course, your card will look prettier because each line of your key card will be in a different color. Now let's move on to creating your stack of statistical assistants.

3. On the front of each card (side without lines) write the full name of one of the inferential statistical tools. Use the broad-tipped, black marker to do this. For example, *Pearson product moment correlation.*

4. Turn the card over and write the information that corresponds to the appropriate category on the key card in the appropriate line using the appropriate color of ink. If you want some assistance with these items use the Critical Thinking Decision Path on page 39 of the textbook. For example, the lined side of the Pearson product moment correlation card would read as follows:

r
IV = 1
DV = 1
IV = at least interval
DV = at least interval relationship (2 variables)
Parametric

ACTIVITY 2

Use the list of terms to complete the items in this activity. Some terms may be used more than once.

ANOVA	Correlation	Nonparametric statistics
Null hypothesis	Parameter	Parametric statistics
Practical significance	Probability	Research hypothesis
Sampling error	Statistic	Statistical significance
Type I error	Type II error	

1. The _____ states that there is no difference between the groups in the study or no association between the variables under study. Its usefulness to a study is that it is the only relationship that can be tested through the use of statistical tools.

2. _____ is an example of the use of _____ .

3. It is impossible to prove that the _____ is true.

4. The tendency for statistics to fluctuate from one sample to another is known as the _____ .

5. The term _____ refers to a characteristics of the population while the term _____ refers to a characteristics of a sample drawn from a population.

6. When investigators are studying the association between variables they often will use statistics that measure _____ .

7. _____ occurs when the investigator does not find statistical significance but a real difference exists in the world. A _____ occurs when the investigator concludes that there is a real (statistically significant) difference but, in reality, there is no difference.

8. The relative frequency of an event in repeated trials under similar conditions is known as _____ and provides the theoretical basis for inferential statistics.

9. A statistically significant finding based on a change of 3 mm/Hg in systolic blood pressure in a sample of healthy individuals likely would have little _____ .

10. _____ refers to those tools used when data are collected at the ordinal or nominal level of measurement.

11. When a finding is tested and found to be unlikely to have happened by chance, the investigators report _____ for that particular finding.

12. When a probability level is calculated as $p < 0.05$ and the investigator had set the alpha level of significance at 0.05, the investigator must reject the _____ and accept the _____ .

13. Identify the components of the following statistical test result. χ^2 (6, n=213) = 33.0, $p < .0001$

   i. χ^2 _____   a. Sample size

   ii. 6   _____   b. Degrees of freedom

   iii. n = 213   _____   c. Chi-square symbol

   iv. 33.0   _____   d. Probability level

   v. $p < .0001$ _____   e. Chi-square test statistic

ACTIVITY 3

We'll walk through the thinking used in inferential statistics with examples from the studies that are included in the text. The researcher's choice of which inferential statistic to use is the result of a fairly long chain of decisions. The decisions begin with the researcher's formulation of the questions that are operating in the clinical setting: If I do this, will it make a difference? If I take this action, will I see a change in the client's status? The decisions regarding research design, sampling strategies, and available data collection instruments follow. All of these decisions lead the researcher to the choice of analytical strategies which would include the choice of inferential statistical techniques.

Let's walk through the Bull, Hansen, and Gross (2000) study found in Appendix A of the textbook while thinking about these decisions.

1.   What was the basic question addressed by Bull, Hansen, and Gross?

2.   Is the research hypothesis written or implied?

3.   Write the null hypothesis for Hypothesis #1.

4.   What function does the null hypothesis serve?

5.   Identify the variables that are identified by the researchers.

  Independent Variable(s):   Dependent Variable(s):

6.   Does the question/research hypothesis/null hypothesis address "differences among groups" or "a relationship between variables"?

7.   How many categories of the independent variable exist?

8.   What level of measurement was used to measure the dependent variable(s)?

9.   Use your "statistical assistant" cards. Which inferential technique do you think was appropriate?

10. Check the study. Is this the one Bull, Hansen, and Gross used?

11. Find the Results section of the study. Within this section find the paragraphs that discuss the outcomes for the caregivers. Read the paragraph that begins "Outcomes for caregivers were also examined. . ." Imagine yourself as the caregiver for an elderly parent or grandparent with heart failure. Based on the information in this paragraph which type of discharge planning would you prefer?

12. Think through and write out the clinical significance of having committed a Type I error in terms of the caregiver's feeling better in the intervention group.

Check your answers with those in Appendix A, Chapter 17.

ACTIVITY 4

Let's practice using the cards. The following items contain information from selected studies. Use the statistical assistant cards you developed in Activity 1 to answer the questions that follow each item.

1. "Of the 280 patient records analyzed, 61.1% (N = 171) met the definition of regular patient, and their clinical outcome data were compared with that of patients who were seen episodically. . . . Overall, regular patients were (a) older (M = 50 years versus 45 years), t (278) = 3.64, p < .001; (b) were more likely to be Hispanic, χ^2 (2, N = 280) = 1.20, p < .01; (c) had both hypertension and diabetes, χ^2 (2, N = 280) = 10.43, p < .05; (d) were nonsmokers, χ^2 (2, N = 280) 19.37, p < .001; (e) were asked about exercise habits, χ^2 (1, N = 279)= 5.60, p < .05; and (f) received pneumococcal, χ^2 (1, N = 280) = 15.65, p < .001, and influenza immunizations, χ^2 (1, N = 280) = 28.56, p < .001." (Bauman, Chang, and Hoebeke, 2002)

   a. What inferential statistics were used with these data?

   b. Explain why the t-statistic was used for the variable of age and the chi-square was used with the other variables.

   c. Both of these statistical procedures were used to compare two groups. What are the groups?

2. Review the data in Figure 1 below which contains self-reported anxiety scores for individuals undergoing colonoscopy with or without music. Each individual reported his/her level of anxiety 4 times: at admission before medication, 5 minutes after medication, at recovery, and at discharge.

Figure 1. Mean State Anxiety by Group During the Colonoscopy

Repeated Measures of ANOVA of Music ($n = 16$) and Nonmusic ($n = 16$) Groups' State Anxiety

Source	df	SS	MS	F	p
Time	1	102.52	102.52	1.87	.18
Group by time	1	87.89	87.89	1.61	.22
Error	30	1643.10	54.77		
Group	1	123.77	123.77	1.80	.19
Error subjects	30	2057.84	68.59		

Smolen D, Topp R, and Singer L (2002). The effect of self-selected music during colonoscopy on anxiety, heart rate, and blood pressure *Appl Nurs Res* 16(2):130.

a. What inferential statistic was used?

b. Why was this the appropriate statistic to use in this situation?

3. The investigators addressed differences between soapsuds and tap water enemas in a group of patients on a liver transplant unit. Table 3 below appears in the report of the study. (Schmelzer, Case, Chappell, and Wright, 2000)

Table 3. Comparison of Enema Instilled, Net Output, PEG Concentration, and Percent of PEG Recovery

	Enema Instilled (g)	Net Output[a] (g)	[PEG][b] (g/L)	PEG Recovery[c]
Tap water group (n = 12)	M: 939 SD: 70 Range: 723 to 980[d]	M: –175.3 SD: 185.6 Range: –556 to +147	M: 1.7 SD: 0.45	68%
Soapsuds group (n = 13)	M: 918 SD: 202 Range: 400 to 976[e]	M: +10.5 SD: 106.1 Range: –205 to +173	M: 1.4 SD: 0.35	72%
Statistical significance (α = .05)	No significant difference (α = .05)	t = –3.039 df = 17 p = .007	No significant difference (α = .05)	No significant difference

[a]Weight of enema returns minus weight of enema instilled.

[b]Concentration of a PEG marker in the enema returns.

[c]Percentage of original polyethylene glycol marker added to the enema that was recovered in the enema returns.

[d]One man retained less than 900 g of tap water; he retained 723 g.

[e]Four people retained less than 900 g of soapsuds enema. Two women received 400 g and 718 g, and two men received 448 g and 794 g of solution.

Schmelzer M, Case P, Chappell SM, and Wright KB (2000). Colonic cleansing, fluid absorption, and discomfort following tap water and soapsuds enemas, *Appl Nurs Res* 13(2):88.

a. How many groups were in this study?

b. What distinguished the groups?

c. The bottom entry of the third column reports "No significant difference (p = .05)." What does this statement mean?

d. The bottom entry in the third column ("Net Output (g)") reports a *t*-statistic and a *p* value of .007. What information does this provide you? Explain why the use of the *t*-statistic was appropriate.

Check your answers with those in Appendix A, Chapter 17.

ACTIVITY 5

Web-Based Activity

Go to www.healthypeople.gov and click on "Leading Health Indicators."

How many leading health indicators are there?

Three reasons were given for selecting these particular health indicators. What are these three reasons?

Now click on "Data" and then on "Major Data Sources." You should be seeing a page that is titled "Part C: Major Data Sources for *Healthy People 2010*." Scroll to the Behavioral Risk Factor Surveillance System and read it. What sentence tells you that inferential statistics are used in this data collection?

POST-TEST

1. The use of a Pearson correlation coefficient and analysis of variance indicates that the variable was measured on which of the following?
   a. Nominal scale
   b. Ordinal scale
   c. Interval or ratio scale

2. Indicate whether the following values are statistically significant or not statistically significant. Use *A* to indicate statistically significant and *B* to indicate not statistically significant. Remember that critical table values are those at the relevant point on the normal distribution curve.

   a. _____ $t = 2.03$, $df = 38$, $p = .01$, critical table value is 2.42

   b. _____ $F_{(2,20)} = 2.67$, $p = .05$, critical table value is 3.49

   c. _____ $\chi^2 = 13.07$, $df = 2$, $p = .05$, critical table value is 5.99

   d. _____ $F_{(3,16)} = 19.20$, $p = .01$, critical table value is 5.29

   e. _____ $t = 6.79$, $df = 58$, $p = .05$, critical table value is 1.67

3.　Use Table 5 from the Chappell, Dickey, and DeLetter study below to answer the last items.

Table 5. Mean Medication Errors per Patient in Residential Care Homes

	Control group mean (n = 46)	Experimental group mean (n = 32)	t-	p
Duplications	.78	.28	1.21	ns
Omissions	2.46	.66	1.87	.06*
Total	3.23	.94	2.22	.03*

From Chappell HW, Dickey C, DeLotta M: The use of medication dispensers in residential care homes, *Family Comm Health* 20(2):48:57, 1997.

a.　Which type of medication error occurred most frequently?

b.　Can you find the arithmetic error in the table?

c.　The experimental group in this study used medication dispensers. Would you advise that this practice be adopted in other residential caregiver situations? Why or why not?

REFERENCES

Bauman LC, Chang M, and Hoebeke R (2002). Clinical outcomes for low-income adults with hypertension and diabetes, *Nurs Res* 51(3):191–198.

Chappell HW, Dickey C, and DeLetter M (1997). The use of medication dispensers in residential care homes, *Family Comm Health* 20(2):48–57.

Schmelzer M, Case P, Chappell SM, and Wright KB (2000). Colonic cleansing, fluid absorption, and discomfort following tap water and soapsuds enemas, *Appl Nurs Res* 13(2):83–91.

Smolen D, Topp R, and Singer L (2002). The effect of self-selected music during colonoscopy on anxiety, heart rate, and blood pressure, *Appl Nurs Res,* 16(2):126–136.

KATHLEEN ROSE-GRIPPA

18

Analysis of Findings

Introduction

As the last sections of a research report, the results and conclusions sections answer the question "So what?" In other words, it is in these two sections that the investigator "makes sense" of the research, critically synthesizes the data, ties them to a theoretical framework, and builds on a body of knowledge. These two sections are a very important part of the research report because they describe the generalizability of the findings and offer recommendations for further research. Well-written, clear, and concise results and conclusions sections provide valuable information for nursing practice. Conversely, poorly written results and conclusions sections will leave a reader bewildered, confused, and wondering how or if the findings are relevant to nursing.

Learning Outcomes

On completion of this chapter, the student should be able to do the following:

- Know the difference between the results sections of a study and the discussion sections of the study.
- Interpret table and figure findings from a research report.
- Describe various generalizations and limitations of a research report.
- Synthesize data and identify implications for nursing.
- Identify recommendations from a research report.

ACTIVITY 1

Knowing what information to look for and where to find it in the Results and Discussions sections of a research report will enable you to interpret the research findings and critique research reports.

1. Identify the section in which the following information from the research report may be found. Put an *A* in the blank space if the information would be found in the Results section and a *B* if the information would be found in the Discussion section.

    a. _____ Tables/figures

    b. _____ Limitations of the study

    c. _____ Data analysis related to the literature review

    d. _____ Inferences or generalization of results

    e. _____ Statistical support or nonsupport of hypotheses

    f. _____ Findings of the hypothesis testing

    g. _____ Information about the statistical tests used to analyze hypotheses

    h. _____ Application of meaning (makes sense) of data analysis

    i. _____ Suggestions for further research

    j. _____ Recommendations for nursing practice

ACTIVITY 2

Tables are an important part of the data analysis component of a study. This activity will focus on tables.

1. Review the following table from Everett, Malarcher, Sharp, Husten, and Giovino (2000). Read the text that address the data in the table. Answer the questions that follow the text excerpt.

Table 2. Prevalence and Odds* of Substance Use Among U.S. High School Students, by Current Tobacco Use Status

	Current Alcohol Use[†]		Current Marijuana Use[§]		Current Cocaine Use[¶]	
	% (CI)**	OR (CI)	% (CI)**	OR (CI)	% (CI)**	OR (CI)
No tobacco use	26.6 (±2.4)	1.0	6.5 (±1.2)	1.0	0.3 (±0.2)	1.0
Cigarettes only	77.2 (±3.6)	9.0 (7.3, 11.0)	48.5 (±3.9)	16.2 (13.4, 19.4)	4.5 (±1.6)	13.1 (6.2, 27.7)
Smokeless tobacco only	65.3 (±14.0)	5.4 (2.9, 10.3)	16.7 (±8.2)	3.1 (1.8, 5.2)	0.1 (±0.2)	0.4 (0.1, 3.1)
Cigars only	68.7 (±5.4)	6.5 (4.7, 8.9)	41.9 (±8.4)	9.7 (6.8, 13.8)	2.0 (±1.8)	7.3 (2.2, 24.2)
Cigarettes and smokeless tobacco only	87.2 (±14.3)	18.4 (5.2, 65.3)	42.9 (±15.1)	12.4 (7.5, 20.5)	13.0 (±8.9)	51.7 (21.8, 122.7)
Cigarettes and cigars only	89.6 (±2.5)	24.3 (18.5, 31.9)	63.4 (±6.2)	26.1 (19.3, 35.4)	7.1 (±1.3)	23.6 (11.9, 46.6)
Smokeless tobacco and cigars only	90.0 (±12.4)	23.1 (5.7, 94.1)	25.8 (±11.7)	5.4 (3.4, 8.6)	7.3 (±7.1)	25.0 (7.2, 86.0)
Cigarettes, smokeless tobacco, and cigars	94.9 (±3.1)	51.8 (28.1, 95.4)	65.5 (±9.2)	30.9 (22.7, 42.1)	20.8 (±5.1)	83.7 (39.3, 178.2)

N = 16,292

*Odds ratios adjusted for gender, race/ethnicity, and grade in school.

[†]Drank alcohol on one or more of the 30 days preceding the survey.

[§]Used marijuana one or more times during the 30 days preceding the survey.

[¶]Used cocaine one or more times during the 30 days preceding the survey.

**95% confidence interval.

Everett SA, Malarcher AM, Sharp DJ, Husten CG, and Giovino, GA (2000). Relationship between cigarette, smokeless tobacco, and cigar use, and other health risk behaviors among U.S. high school students, *Journal of School Health* 70(6):236. Reprinted with permission. American School Health Association, Kent, Ohio.

Current Tobacco Use and Other Substance Use

Generally, students who used tobacco were significantly more likely than nonusers to report current use of alcohol, marijuana, and cocaine (Table 2). The only exception occurred among students who used only smokeless tobacco; the prevalence of cocaine use did not differ from nontobacco users. Students who used all three tobacco products had the highest prevalence of alcohol use (94.9%; OR = 51.8), marijuana use (65.5%; OR = 30.9), and cocaine use (20.8%; OR = 83.7). Among students who used only one tobacco product, the odds of other drug use were the greatest among cigarette users and lowest among smokeless tobacco users. The likelihood of alcohol and cocaine use increased as the number of tobacco products the student used increased. In contrast, the odds of marijuana use were significantly higher among users of cigarettes only (OR = 16.2) than among users of both smokeless tobacco and cigars (OR = 5.4).

a. Does the information in the table meet the criteria for a table as described on page 369 of the textbook? Explain.

b. Which group was most likely to be currently using cocaine?

c. Of the students who used only one of the three possible tobacco products, what was the other substance most commonly used and which group reported the greatest use of this substance?

ACTIVITY 3

Collect demographic data on the people in your research class. You can decide what data you want to collect but common variables would be age, gender, eye color, hair color (current or underlying), etc. Once the data have been collected, work in groups of no less than three but no more than five and create a table that displays these data. Exchange tables with another group. Critique each other's tables with the intent of improving them.
    Criteria to consider:

a. Are data summaries included rather than all of the raw data?

b. Is the title clear? Do you know what data are being presented without needing to read the text?

c. Are the columns and rows appropriately labeled?

d. Other criteria you want to include? Your instructor suggests?

ACTIVITY 4

This activity will give you some practice in the interpretation of research articles. Read the Mahon, Yarcheski, and Yarcheski (2000) article in Appendix C of the textbook and answer the following items.

1.   The following items pertain to Table 1 of the article.

   a.   What is the meaning of the "(N = 141)" on this table?

   b.   Which variable would you suspect is the most heterogeneous?

   c.   What data did you use to answer item b?

2.   Look at Table 2.

   a.   Name the variable pairs for which there were statistically significant correlations.

   b.   How does the relationship between symptom patterns and trait anger differ from the relationship between well-being and trait anger?

3.   Go to the study by Bull, Hansen, and Gross (2000) in Appendix A of the textbook.

   a.   How many *individuals* are represented by the numbers in Table 1?

   b.   Who were the subjects in Table 4?

   c.   What was the finding regarding continuity of information between the intervention group and the control group at the 2 months postdischarge interview?

Check your answers with those in Appendix A, Chapter 18.

ACTIVITY 5

Web-Based Activity

Go to www.google.com. Type "analysis" in the search box. Scroll down and look at all of the web sites that use "analysis" in their description. There were 39,000,000 hits on the day I completed this exercise. Look through a few pages (usually 10 sites on each page). On a scale of 1 to 10, where would you place the value of using the word "analysis" as a search term when looking for studies relevant to nursing? Play with modifiers of "analysis" and see if you can get some useful information from this search.

POST-TEST

1. When a research hypothesis is supported through testing, it may be assumed that the hypothesis was which of the following?
   a. Proved
   b. Accepted
   c. Rejected
   d. Disconfirmed

2. Limitations of a study describe its weaknesses.
   True   False

3. The Results section of a research study includes all the following except:
   a. Hypothesis testing results.
   b. Tables and figures.
   c. Statistical test description.
   d. Limitations of the study.

4. Unsupported hypotheses mean that the study is of little value in generating knowledge.
   True   False

5. Tables in research reports should meet all of the following criteria *except*:
   a. Clear, concise tables.
   b. Restate the text narrative.
   c. Economize the text.
   d. Supplement the text narrative.

6. The discussion section provides opportunity for the investigator to do all of the following *except*:
   a. Describe implications from the research results.
   b. Relate the results to the literature review.
   c. Make generalizations to large populations of subjects.
   d. Suggest areas for further research.

7. Hypothesis testing is described in the discussion section of the research report.
   True   False

The answers to the post-test are on the textbook's web site. Please check with your instructor for these answers.

REFERENCES

Everett SA, Malarcher AM, Sharp DJ, Husten CG, and Giovino GA (2000). Relationship between cigarette, smokeless tobacco, and cigar use, and other health risk behaviors among U.S. high school students. *Journal of School Health* 70(6):234–240.

Mahon NE, Yarcheski A, and Yarcheski TJ (2000). Positive and negative outcomes of anger in early adolescents, *Res Nurs & Hlth* 23:17–24.

KATHLEEN ROSE-GRIPPA

19

Evaluating Quantitative Research

Introduction

Now is the time for you to put together all of the pieces that you have studied throughout this book. Read through the studies and the written critiques that are part of Chapter 19 in the textbook.

A useful way of doing this is as follows:

1. Read the research report from beginning to end. Do not stop to puzzle over this particular piece or that particular section. Just start at the beginning and read to the end. This will give you an impression of the article as a whole.
2. Read through the critiquing guidelines found in Table 19-1 of the textbook.
3. Read the journal article again. This time jot down any thoughts that might occur to you while reading. The margins of the book or those of the copy of the journal article are easy places to note thoughts that you want to review again.
4. Now go through the article section by section. Read the questions from Table 19-1, then read the relevant section of the research report. Answer the questions. The answers to these questions will become the working draft of the written critique.
5. Now write in narrative style the critique you have just finished thinking through. Be careful with your use of language. Do not be brutal, but do raise any questions that you have.

Learning Outcomes

On completion of this chapter, the student should be able to do the following:

- Practice thinking through a critique.
- Practice writing a critique.

ACTIVITY 1

The exercise for this chapter is to practice thinking through a critique. The two critiques presented in the text will give you a sense of style, length, and flow. After you have read them, read the Mahon, Yarcheski, and Yarcheski (2000) study in Appendix C of the text. Read as though you were going to write a critique of the study. Use the steps listed above. Write a first draft of a critique.

1. Problem Statement and Purpose

2. Hypotheses or Research Questions

3. Review of Literature

4. Theoretical Framework

5. Research Design

6. Sample

7. Legal and Ethical Issues

8. Data Collection Methods

9. Reliability and Validity

10. Analysis of Findings

11. Conclusions, Implications, and Recommendations

The answers in Appendix A, Chapter 19 will not provide you with a written critique, but they will give you the answers to the questions listed in the critiquing guidelines table in Chapter 19.

Note: There is no post-test for this chapter… Enjoy the break!

KATHLEEN ROSE-GRIPPA

20

Use of Research in Practice

Introduction

Research is important to the clinician as a means to support current practice or to provide data to support a practice change. When using research to support or change practice, the clinician should consider two main aspects. First, what interventions provide the best patient outcomes? If there is no difference in patient outcomes when considering two or more interventions, then cost, in both dollars and time, should also be considered. Second, if there is research support for a practice change, what process should the clinician follow for implementation?

Learning Outcomes

On completion of this chapter, the student should be able to do the following:

- Interpret a summary table to determine recommendations for practice.
- Identify organizational forces that affect research utilization.
- Evaluate an individual research study for its potential for utilization in the student's clinical setting.

ACTIVITY 1

This activity is to help you gain familiarity with the terms and concepts associated with using research in practice.

1. Name the first nurse to use data to improve health care.

2. Match the term in Column B to its definition in Column A. Each term is used only once.

<table>
<tr><td align="center">**Column A**</td><td align="center">**Column B**</td></tr>
<tr><td>a. _____ Use of research findings to improve nursing care</td><td>A. Dissemination of findings</td></tr>
<tr><td></td><td>B. Research utilization</td></tr>
<tr><td>b. _____ Analysis of data collected for the purpose of answering questions or testing hypotheses</td><td>C. Evidence-based practice</td></tr>
<tr><td></td><td>D. Conduct of research</td></tr>
<tr><td>c. _____ Reporting of research findings at scientific conferences or through articles in journals</td><td>E. CURN and the Orange County Research Utilization in Nursing Activity</td></tr>
<tr><td>d. _____ Demonstration projects in use of research in nursing care</td><td></td></tr>
<tr><td>e. _____ Conscience and judicious use of the best evidence in the care of clients</td><td></td></tr>
</table>

3. Explain the difference between a "problem-focused trigger" and a "knowledge-focused trigger" in evidence-based practice.

4. The steps to put evidence-based practice into place are listed below. They are NOT in the conceptually correct sequence. Put a "1" next to the event that is to occur first and an "11" next the last activity in the sequence. Number each of the items between 1 and 11 with the number indicating its place in the sequence.

   a. _____ Critique the research studies relevant to the topic.

   b. _____ Synthesize the findings in the research.

   c. _____ Selection of a topic.

   d. _____ Review theoretical and clinical articles on the topic.

   e. _____ Review existing EBP guidelines.

f. _____ Decide to change practice.

g. _____ Form a team.

h. _____ Recommend changes in practice.

i. _____ Choose a mechanism for grading the evidence.

j. _____ Find relevant literature.

k. _____ Classify articles by type.

5. You have determined that a change in practice is warranted. Explain the three most important actions you need to take to implement the change in practice.

a.

b.

c.

Check your answers with those in Appendix A, Chapter 20.

ACTIVITY 2

Time to think. Think of some clinical concern you have. It may be a treatment that you think caused more pain than was needed, a problem with the administration of some medication, a concern about ambulation assistance, etc. Pick something in which you are interested. Write down the topic.

Topic of interest to me is:

Now go to at least three of the following sites and discover what is available. List the title(s) of relevant resources.

http://www.guideline.gov
http://www.ampainsoc.org
http://www.ons.org
http://www.aacn.org
http://www.awhonn.org
http://www.nursing.uiowa.edu/gnirc

http://www.update.cochrane.co.uk
http://www.updateusa.com
http://www.cche.net
http://www.acponline.com
http://www.ovid.com
http://www.thoracic.org

Did you find articles that addressed your topic? Have you read any of these articles? Do the titles read as though they might contain some good practice information? If you are on a site that allows you access to the article itself, open it up and look at it. Is the information consistent with what you have been practicing in relevant situations?

Discuss with your colleagues the success or lack of success that you had in finding EBP guidelines for the topic in which you were interested. What could you do to improve the situation?

ACTIVITY 3

This is another thinking activity. Again, think of a topic of clinical interest. You may continue with the one you used in the previous activity or you may change topics. Find three research studies that address the topic. Remember that it is rare to find the topic phrased exactly how you have written it. You may have to look for specific keywords. Use the CINAHL electronic database.

Once you have the articles, complete a table comparable to that in Figure 20-5 in the textbook. Now look over that information and based on these three articles, what would you conclude about practice in this particular area?

ACTIVITY 4

Read each of the articles found in the appendices of the textbook. Address each of the items in relation to each of the studies.

1. Indicate for each article whether utilization of the results would be considered conceptual [c] or decision driven [d].

    a. _____ Bull, Hansen, and Gross (2000)

    b. _____ Cohen and Ley (2000)

    c. _____ Mahon, Yarcheski, and Yarcheski (2000)

    d. _____ LoBiondo-Wood, Williams, Kouzekanani, and McGhee (2000)

2. Think about each study. Using the Iowa model (Figure 20-2, p. 416, in the text) or the Rosswurm model (Figure 20-3, p. 418, in the text) how important would you consider the application of each study in your clinical setting?

    a. What is the topic of each study?

       Bull, Hansen, and Gross

       Cohen and Levy

       Mahon, Yarcheski, and Yarcheski

       LoBiondo-Wood et al.

    b. What priority would each topic have in terms of your interests in nursing?

       Bull, Hansen, and Gross

       Cohen and Levy

       Mahon, Yarcheski, and Yarcheski

       LoBiondo-Wood et al.

    c. What would be the magnitude of the topic in your setting, e.g. would the topic affect a few or many clinical areas? Is the problem one that is high frequency? High risk? High cost?

    d. Assume there is a rich body of research on each topic that supports the findings of the studies in the appendices. How might practice change?

e. Again, assuming there is a strong research base, would your setting be ready to change in the direction(s) you suggested in item d, or are there sensitive issues to consider and address?

Check your answers with those in Appendix A, Chapter 20.

ACTIVITY 5

Web-Based Activity

Go to www.cinahl.com and click on "Evidence-based Practice Web Sites" and click on "Health Web." Read through some of this site. Which group of healthcare professionals would most likely find this site useful?

Go back to the CINAHL home page. Click on "nursing" and then on "General and Special Topics." Look through the topics that pop up. Are any of them relevant to your preferred area of practice?

POST-TEST

1. Name four demonstration projects of research utilization:

   a.

   b.

   c.

   d.

2. List six of the eight elements of essential information to include for each study on a summary table:

   a.

   b.

   c.

   d.

   e.

   f.

3. Define the following terms in respect to research utilization:

   a. Change champion

   b. Core group

   c. Outcome data

   d. Process data

   e. Organizational climate

4. Discuss at least three ways the nurse executive can encourage research utilization.

   a.

   b.

   c.

5. Clinical articles can provide the basis for a practice change.
    True   False

6. If a research study has any flaws, it cannot be used to support a practice change.
    True   False

7. Cost is as important as clinical outcomes when considering a practice change.
    True   False

8. Research utilization is an important aspect of the staff nurse role.
    True   False

The answers to the post-test are on the textbook's web site. Please check with your instructor for these answers.

REFERENCES

Bull MJ, Hansen HE, and Gross CR (2000). A professional-patient partnership model of discharge planning with elders hospitalized with heart failure, *Appl Nurs Res* 13(1):19–28.

Cohen MZ and Ley CD (2000). Bone marrow transplantation: the battle for hope in face of fear, *Oncol Nurs Forum* 27(3):473–480.

LoBiondo-Wood G, Williams L, Kouzekanani K, and McGhee C (2000). Family adaptation to a child's transplant: pretransplant phase, *Progress in Transplantation* 10(2):81–87.

Mahon NE, Yarcheski A, and Yarcheski T (2000). Positive and negative outcomes of anger in early adolescents, *Res Nurs Health* 23:17–24.

Appendix A
Answers to Activities

CHAPTER 1

Activity 1
1. c
2. b
3. d
4. a
5. f
6. e

Activity 2
1. D
2. B
3. C
4. D
5. A
6. B
7. A
8. C
9. B

Activity 3
1. a. PhD, RN; PhD, RN; PhD
   b. PhD, RN; RN, MN
   c. unknown; unknown; unknown
   d. PhD, RN; MSN, RN; PhD; PhD
2. a. A = Yes; B = Yes; C = Unknown; D = Yes
   b. **Appendix A:** Authors one (Margaret Bull), two (Helen Hansen), and three (Gross) are doctorally prepared and would obviously be more than qualified to design and implement the study.
   Appendix B: Marlene Cohen, the first author, is a doctorally prepared nurse who has the educational preparation to design and conduct research. The second author, Cathaleen Ley, is a master's prepared nurse who is also a doctoral student. She also appears to be appropriate to design and implement a study.
   Appendix C: Although no educational preparation is mentioned for the three authors, authors one (Noreen Mahon) and two (Adela Yarcheski) are professors in the College of Nursing and author three (Thomas Yarcheski) is an Associate Professor in the Department of Professional Management. Based on their positions at the universities, I would state that these authors appear to be appropriate to design and implement a study.

Appendix D: Geri LoBiondo-Wood, the first author, is a doctorally prepared nurse who has the educational preparation to design and conduct research. The second author, Laurel Williams, is a master's prepared nurse, whose role is not stated. Authors three (Kamiar Kouzekanani) and four (Charles McGhee) are also doctorally prepared and are able to design and conduct research.

c. **Appendix A:** The Bull, Hansen, and Gross study was funded by the Retirement Research Foundation of Chicago.

Appendix B: No mention is made of funding sources in the Cohen and Ley article.

Appendix C: No mention is made of funding sources in the Mahon, Yarcheski, and Yarcheski article.

Appendix D: The LoBiondo et al. study was funded by the National Institute of Nursing Research, National Institutes of Health, Washington, DC.

Activity 4

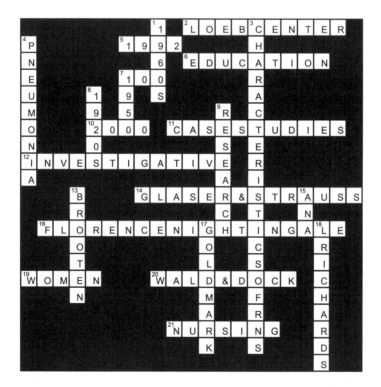

Activity 5

a. Continuing to conduct research on the topic of abuse in women.
b. Developing theoretical perspectives that provide a basis for interventions.
c. Conducting synthesis conferences discussing the area of abuse of women.
d. Using nursing research studies to assist in legislative change.

Activity 6

1. In order to base my practice on scientific evidence gained through research, I must first understand the research process. Then I need to know how to critique research in order to decide whether particular studies and their results have enough merit to change my practice.
2. Depth in nursing science will occur when a sufficient number of nurse researchers replicate and have consistent findings in a substantive area of inquiry. It is important that each study builds on prior studies, adding new variables or questions as the need arises.
3. Because my area of practice is psychiatric/mental health nursing with an emphasis on chemical dependency, I would like research findings demonstrating that nursing interventions related to "knowledge deficit regarding addiction" have an effect on the outcome of increased sobriety time for the addict or alcoholic.

CHAPTER 2

Activity 1

1. Rational
2. Active; inner
3. Writer of what is being read
4. Nursing
5. Three (or four)

Activity 2

1. b
2. b
3. a
4. b
5. a
6. a

Activity 3

1. a. Preliminary understanding
   b. Comprehensive understanding
   c. Analysis understanding
   d. Synthesis understanding
2. a. Read the article for the fourth time
   b. Review the notes you have written on your copy of the article
   c. Summarize study in own words
   d. Complete one handwritten 5 x 8 card per study
   e. Staple the summary to the top of copied article

Activity 4

1. No
2. No

3. Yes (The exact term correlational is not used; however, if you look at the definition of correlation in the glossary, it states that correlation is "the degree of association between the two variables.") The authors imply that the research problem is relationship between family variables of stress, coping, social support, perception of stress, and family adaptation.
4. No (Although the term *convenience* could be used appropriately to describe this sample.)
5. Yes (Instruments used include the: 1) Family Inventory of Life Events and Changes, 2) Coping Health Inventory for Parents, 3) Norbeck Social Support Questionnaire, 4) Parent Perception of Uncertainty Scale, 5) Profile of Mood States, and 6) McMaster Family Assessment Device) (p. 482 of the textbook).
6. Yes (pp. 482-483)
7. Yes (p. 483) Summary: I would categorize this study as quantitative. It meets 4 of the 7 criteria listed. It is not experimental or quasiexperimental (two of the specific types of quantitative designs that are usually the only ones that would include using the terms hypotheses, control, and treatment group). Instead it is nonexperimental.

Activity 5

I would go to the reference section and locate the article by Freeberg which is located in the *Journal of Psychosocial Nursing and Mental Health Services.* The other selections are found in books. I would then go to the library or an online source, find the article or book, and photocopy the part needed. I would probably look at the Izard (1977, 1991) references first since the titles, *Human Emotion* and *the Psychology of Emotions,* relate to the emotion of anger. It is not uncommon to need to seek out primary and secondary sources from the reference list to critically analyze an article.

CHAPTER 3

Activity 1
1. e
2. b
3. d
4. a
5. c

Activity 2
1. Yes; Yes; Yes; Yes
2. No; No; Yes; Yes
3. Yes; No; Yes; Yes

Activity 3
1. a. CRTs
   b. Birth defects
2. a. Birth defects
   b. Independence/dependence conflicts
3. a. White wine

     b.   Serum cholesterol level
4. a.   Type of recording
     b.   Patient care
5. a.   Profession (MD or RN)
     b.   Extended-role concept of RNs
6. a.   Sex, age, height, weight
     b.   Physiologic outcomes

Activity 4

1. Hr, DH
2. Hr, DH
3. RQ
4. Hr, DH
5. Hr, NDH
6. RP

Activity 5

1. RQ: Does the use of CRTs by pregnant women influence the incidence of birth defects?
    Ho: The use of CRTs by pregnant women has no effect on the incidence of birth defects.
2. DH: As is in the chapter.
    NDH: There is a difference in the number of independence/dependence conflicts between individuals with and without birth defects.
    Hr: As is.
    RQ: Do individuals with birth defects have a higher incidence of independence/dependence conflicts than those without birth defects?
    Ho: There is no difference in incidence of independence/dependence conflicts between individuals with and without birth defects.
3. DH: There is a positive relationship between daily moderate consumption of white wine and serum cholesterol levels.
    NDH: Daily moderate consumption of white wine influences serum cholesterol levels.
    Hr: There is a relationship between daily moderate consumption of white wine and serum cholesterol levels.
    RQ: As is.
    Ho: There is no relationship between daily moderate consumption of white wine and serum cholesterol levels.

Activity 6

1. a.   Yes
     b.   Yes; IV-SPID; DV-dressing independence
     c.   Yes
     d.   Yes
     e.   Yes
     f.   Yes
     g.   Yes
2. a.   Yes
     b.   Yes
     c.   Yes

    d. Yes
    e. Yes
    f. Yes
    g. Yes

Activity 7

1. a. There is probably not enough time for the student to design and conduct this study. It will take a considerable amount of time to conceptualize this problem and would be a more appropriate study for a doctoral thesis where a student usually has 3 years to resolve a problem. The first year of doctoral study, the student could work on refining the problem in design classes, and then have a full 1 to 2 years to conduct the study, analyze the data, and complete the write-up.
   b. This is difficult to answer based on the information given in the brief scenario. Because the nurse has identified it as a problem, I would assume she or he is aware of a unit where this change is occurring; whether the nurse would be able to gain access to that unit to conduct research is an unknown until she or he sends a letter and asks permission of the setting and the setting's Institutional Review Board.
   c. The lack of experience of the researcher is probably the greatest impediment to conducting this study. It will take a very experienced and knowledgeable researcher to determine which variables to study and to develop a study design that will give meaningful answers to this question. This is probably why the definitive study in this area has not yet been done.
   d. I do not foresee any ethical issues inherent in conducting this study.
2. a. Yes
   b. This could be a very significant study for the practice of nursing. It brings into study the relationship between level of practitioner and quality of care. It could also address economic considerations of care; e.g., is it less expensive to use caregivers who cost less to employ or more cost effective to employ caregivers who can provide more complete care?

Activity 8

The problem statement poses the question the researcher is asking. The hypothesis attempts to answer the question posed by the research problem. The problem statement does not predict a relationship between two or more variables.

CHAPTER 4

Activity 1

1. Research
2. Education
3. Research; practice
4. Theory

Activity 2

1. f
2. c

3. a
4. e
5. d
6. c
7. b

Activity 3
1. D
2. C
3. D
4. D
5. C
6. D

Activity 4
(*Note:* Choose from any of the following scholarly nursing journals for the five correct answers.) *Advances in Nursing, AORN Journal, Applied Nursing Research, Archives of Psychiatric Nursing, Computers in Nursing, Heart & Lung, Holistic Nursing Practice, Image: Journal of Nursing Scholarship, Journal of Professional Nursing, Journal of Nursing Education, NACOG, Nurse Educator, Nursing Diagnosis, Nursing & Health Care, Nursing Research, Nursing Science Quarterly, Research in Nursing & Health, Scholarly Inquiry for Nursing Practice,* and *Western Journal of Nursing Research.*

Activity 5
1. a. Background
    b. No title given. (*Note:* Literature review begins after the key points.)
2. a. Yes, these authors noted that previous studies have not addressed factors that influence caregiver participation in planning for discharge.
    b. Yes, these authors uncover a gap in prior research. They note that although there has been much research on the patient's perspective of BMT, all but one informant had allogeneic transplants, not autologous transplants.
3. Yes, the majority of the references in this article are current, ranging from 1992–1997. It does read like a well-designed research proposal. The first cited research on the topic was cited in 1966, in which an evaluating approach of medical care was studied from which the authors' conceptual framework for the study is based. Studies completed in the early-to-mid 1990s discuss the variables and outcomes that had been examined in elder discharge planning along with instruments to assess. Thus, the authors identified gaps in the literature of factors that influence caregiver participation in discharge planning. When this research was initiated, new variables were identified to study outcomes for elders and caregivers who participate in a professional-patient partnership model.

Activity 6
1. a. S
    b. P
    c. S
    d. S

e. P
f. P
g. P
2. False
3. False
4. True
5. True
6. b, MEDLINE does not contain all nursing references like CINAHL does.
7. True
8. True
9. False

Activity 7
1. D; P
2. D; P
3. D; P
4. D; P
5. D; S

Activity 8
1. What is the source of the material? (*Note:* Look at the last term in the URL address to find the organizational name [it is three letters long]; possibilities include: *com* for commercial organization, *edu* for educational institution, *gov* for government body, *int* for international organization, *mil* for U.S. military, *net* for networking organization, and *org* for anything else. I would feel most comfortable with information gathered from an *edu* or *gov* source, such as www.ncbi.nlm.nih.gov that takes me to the Pub Med Query source for MEDLINE at the U.S. National Library of Medicine or from a respected international honor society, such as Sigma Theta Tau International at http://www.stti.iupui.edu/library/.)
2. Is the source a well-respected medical or nursing institution or a federal agency, or is the source an individual putting out his/her own opinion? Critique the source.
3. Are the name(s) of the researcher or researchers and her/his/their degrees given?
4. Is there a mechanism given to obtain further information about the study or the information presented?
5. Is enough data given in the web publication to make a critical analysis about the material, such as the analysis I would make about a research article using the critiquing criteria in the textbook? (*Note:* Remember, in a referred, professional journal usually three independent nursing experts in the field have reviewed the article in a blind review process to determine that this material merits publication.)

CHAPTER 5

Activity 1
1. Inductive thinking: moves from the particular to the general (or conclusions are developed from specific observations)
    Deductive thinking: moves from the general to the particular (or predictions are developed from known relationships)

2. a. Inductive
    b. Deductive
3. (Observations will vary.) If you were able to write a general statement about "headache pain," you used inductive thinking and probably wrote something like:

    X (grimacing) X (rubbing temples) X (grumpy) = indications of headache pain.

    If you were unable to write a general statement, a reason could be that you do not know anyone who has headaches, so you do not have a database.

Activity 2
1. a. Learned helplessness, self-esteem, depression, health practices, homeless (*Note:* You would also be correct if you listed women.)
    b. Illness, uncertainty, stress, coping, emotional well-being, clinical drug trial
    c. Social support, intervention, pregnancy, pregnancy outcome, lower income, African American
    d. Violent behavior, nonviolent behavior, behavior, vulnerable, inner-city youths
    e. Verbal abuse, staff nurses, physicians, stress coping (*Note:* Prevalence and consequences may also be listed as consequences especially if you think of them as capturing an idea.)
2. a. "Beauty" is a concept. "Nursing diagnosis" is a construct.
    b. "Beauty" and "nursing diagnosis" are similar in that both describe an abstraction. Both terms describe some notion that people want to be able to discuss, think about, or use without spending hours describing what is meant.
    c. The terms are different in one important dimension. "Beauty" is a concept that all people recognize, although the precise characteristics of beauty may vary from person to person. The construct "nursing diagnosis," is an abstraction that has been created by a specific discipline to explain a concept unique to that discipline. All disciplines, especially researchers within a given discipline, create constructs to structure their world of study.
3. There are no "correct" answers for this question. Rather, the thinking that you do to reach a consensus is the "correct answer." An argument could be made for the following as constructs: illness uncertainty, social support intervention, and verbal abuse.
4. a. Answers will vary.
    b. Answers will vary.

Activity 3
1. The two major concepts are discharge planning and patient/caregiver outcome measures. Each of these was operationally defined as follows:
    Discharge planning: One of two types—usual discharge planning procedures or a professional-patient partnership model of discharge planning.
    Patient outcomes: Defined as perceived health, client satisfaction caregiver's response to caregiving, and resource use. These definitions are further defined in Table 2, which lists the instruments used.
2. The concepts of this study were hope and fear. Given the qualitative nature of this study, precise definitions would not be expected. The intent of this study is to more clearly articulate the concept.

3. The major concepts in this study are trait anger, state anger, general well-being, symptom patterns, vigor, and inclination to change.
   Trait anger: Defined as responses to items on the Spielberger Trait Anger Scale that assess how angry one generally feels.
   State anger: Defined as responses to items on the Spielberger State Anger Scale that assess how angry one is feeling right now.
   General well-being: Defined as responses to items on the Adolescent General Well-Being Questionnaire that assess the social, physical, and mental dimensions of well-being.
   Symptom patterns: Defined as responses to items on the Symptom Pattern Scale that measure physical, psychological, and psychosomatic manifestations of psychological distress.
   Vigor: Defined as responses to items on the Vigor subscale of the Profile of Mood States that assesses vigor.
   Inclination to change: Defined as responses to items on the change subscale of the Personality-Research Form-E that assess inclination to change.
4. The major concepts in this study are pile-up, existing and new resources, perception of stressors, and adaptation.
   Pile-up: Defined as family strains and as responses to items on the Family Inventory of Life Events and Changes that assess family stress variables with the ability to assess the pile-up events.
   Existing and new resources: Defined as social support and coping. Social support is defined as responses to items on the Norbeck Social Support questionnaire that evaluates a person's social support network. Coping is defined as responses to items on the Coping Health Inventory for Parents that assess parent's coping responses in the management of family life when a child is seriously ill.
   Perception of stressor: Defined as responses to items on the Parent Perception of Uncertainty Scale that assesses a parent's perception of uncertainty as a stress. Also defined as responses to the Profile of Mood States that assesses a person's level of mood and subjective affect.
   Family adaptation: Defined as responses to items on the McMaster's Family Assessment Device that assesses family functioning and used to measure family adaptation.

Activity 4
1. a. 4
   b. 5
   c. 6
   d. 4
   e. 5 or 3
   f. 3
   g. 6
   h. 1
   i. 2
2. a. Anger
   b. i. Anger is a major concern of early adolescents and it has not been studied much in this population.
      ii. There is a lack of studies on positive outcomes of anger in early adolescents.
      iii. Trait anger and state anger are defined by Spielberger and colleagues.
      iv. Personality traits have an impact on the way people are predisposed to behave or act in a certain way.
      v. Described variables in model and how they relate to one another.
      vi. Anger can be exhibited as symptom patterns in adolescents.
   c. Deductive

d.   Yes
e.   Conceptual model

Activity 5

Critiquing Grid

	Well Done	OK	Needs Help	Not Applicable
1. Theoretical rationale was clearly identified (Could I find it?)	B; C; M; L			
2. The information in the theoretical component matches what the researchers are studying.	B; C; M; L			
3. Concepts:				
a. Conceptual definition(s) found	M; L	B		C
b. Conceptual definition(s) clear	M; L	B		C
c. Operational definition(s) found	M; L	B		C
d. Operational definition(s) clear	M; L	B		C
4. Enough literature was reviewed:				
a. For an expert in the area.	B; M; L		C	
b. For a nurse with some knowledge.	B; M; L	C		
c. For a nurse reading outside of area of specialty or interest.	B; M; L	C		
5. The researcher's thinking:				
a. Can be followed through theoretical material to hypotheses or questions.	B; M; L			C
b. Makes sense.	B; M; L	C		
6. Relationships among propositions clearly stated.	B; M; L			C
7. Theory:				
a. Borrowed				B; C; M; L
b. Concepts/data related to nursing	B; C; L	M		
8. Findings related back to theoretical base. (I can find each concept from the theory section discussed in the "Results" section of the report.)	B; C; M; L			

(*Note:* As you see, it is not easy to make unequivocal statements about every criterion. Some criteria do not fit one study as well as they fit another study. The use of a grid like the one above is a start in your critical thinking. It makes sure that you have addressed the same areas for each study. You then have to put this information together with your evaluation of the other pieces of the study to make the final critical judgment of the quality of the specific study.)

CHAPTER 6

Activity 1
1. a. Empirical knowledge: Factual knowledge based upon scientific evidence.
   b. Moral knowledge: Allows nurses to look at morality embedded in diverse situations and recognize how these perspectives flavor reactions and direct the interventions selected.
   c. Personal knowing: The lived experience the nurse brings to the nursing situation or what each nurse brings to a client situation.
   d. Aesthetic knowing: Use of intuition and empathy to understand clients' uniqueness. It bypasses the usual linear process of thinking and challenges one to see the multitude of possibilities in a given situation.
2. a. Go to the "Philosophy and History" http://www.uwm.edu/~brodg/philos.htm web site. Here is an example of what your paragraph about a selected philosopher might look. Karl Popper was the philosopher selected. A web site used to find much more extensive information about him was http://plato.stanford.edu/entries/popper/#Life.

   　　Karl Popper's (1902–1994) leading philosophical perspective had to do with methodological views called Falsification. Falsification is the idea that science advances by unjustified or unfounded presumptions that are then liberally criticized by the scientific world. Theories that are falsifiable can expand knowledge by improving our control about errors in judgment as to what is true or false about the world. Theories that are unfalsifiable are only problems to clear thinking and act like log jams in the stream of knowledge. Popper thought that while a theory could be unscientific (unfalsifiable), it could still be enlightening and able to become falsified or scientific with further refinement. Popper thought that a major problem in the philosophy of science was determining differences between what is scientific and what comprises nonscience. From his perspective, a genuine test of a scientific theory is an attempt to refute or falsify it. Although a theory has stood for a long while and appears to be good science, it is still possible that error exists and at some later time the theory may be falsified.

   b. Go to "Ereignis" http://webcom.com/paf/ereignis.html and learn about Heidegger. Another site about this philosopher is a link to the Encarta web site http://www.connect.net/ron/heid/html.

   　　Martin Heidegger (1889–1976), a German philosopher, developed the ideas of existential phenomenology. This philosophical perspective explores the essential question: What is it, to be? Humans are continually affected by the world they live in and struggle with time, objects, daily routines, and the behavior of others. Heidegger's most influential work is entitled *Being and Time* (1927, translated 1962). He believed that the existence of physical body came before the fundamental nature of self, but at some point a being becomes aware of its own existence and a new essence is formed. Human being is comprised of concern, being-toward death, existence, and moods.

Activity 2

a. Epistemology: A branch of philosophy that deals with what we know as truth or knowledge and includes its origins, limits, and nature.

b. Ontology: A branch of philosophy that studies the nature of being or existence.

c. Context: The place where something occurs and can include physical place, cultural beliefs, and life experiences.

d. Perceived paradigm: The basis of most qualitative research. The goal of this research is to explore meanings related to multiple realities. Ontology and context are important aspects of exploring meanings and realities.

e. Received paradigm: The basis of most quantitative research. The goal of this research is to use statistical measures to describe, explain, predict, and ultimately to control the variables of interest.

Activity 3

Your answer may be different, but here is an example of some differences.

If pain management associated with cancer were to be considered using the received paradigm, the approaches might be to consider and measure the physiological nature of pain mechanisms. In this case, it is likely that the investigator might choose a design with several control groups to study the efficacy of various drugs or treatments. The researcher may choose to obtain a large group of participants for the study that represent a mix of gender, races, ages, or cultures to see if the treatment provides equal effectiveness in managing pain. The goal of this research might be to ascertain whether one treatment is more effective than another. However, if pain management were to be studied using the perceived paradigm, the number of study participants may be small and they may be homogeneous in nature. This study would be considerate of the participants' values relevant to various experiences. The goal of this study might be to identify the realities of the lived experience of cancer pain in order to better understand what patients and families experience when treatment is not therapeutic.

Activity 4

1. a. Grounded theory: A research method that enables the investigator to discover a theory from systematically obtained data. The data comes from the observations of the participants being studied. The purpose of this form of research is to generate theory.

    b. Case study: A research method that provides an in-depth description of the phenomena of interest to the investigator. Data for case studies may come from a variety of sources. This research method provides a way to study complex phenomena that are poorly understood.

    c. Phenomenological research: A research method that examines naturalistic experiences as they are lived and understood as reality by human beings. Researchers examine phenomena that are of special interest to nursing. The goal of this type of research is to understand experience from the perspective of those having the experience.

    d. Ethnographic research: A research method initially developed by anthropologists to study the ways human beings react within or experience a cultural setting. The goal is to combine the emic (insider) with the etic (outsider) perspective. Nurses have adapted this method to study health and illness within a variety of cultural contexts.

2. A. Grounded theory: The grounded theory approach to research seems well-suited to the need for nursing's understandings about social behaviors. Unstructured interview or conversation with a purpose is often used in this form of research. Data are analyzed by using abstract categories until saturation is reached or no new information is being discovered.
    B. Case study: Case studies often involve in-depth interviews with participants and key informants, medical record reviews, observation, and excerpts from patients' personal writings and diaries. Life histories can serve as a way to understand a person or phenomena of concern over a long period of time. Case study designs must have five components: the research question(s), its propositions, its unit(s) of analysis, a determination of how the data are linked to the propositions, and criteria to interpret the findings (Yin, 1994).
    C. Phenomenological research: Phenomenology entails listening and truly hearing what persons are saying and understanding the lived experience from their perspective. This type of research requires an attitude of radical openness and extreme attentiveness to the world we live in.
    D. Ethnographic research: The goal of ethnographic research is to look for patterns, themes, connections, and relationships that have meanings for the persons involved. Questions of interest in the ethnographic process are: What is this? What's happening in this subculture? Gaining access to data in an ethnographic study usually entails identifying a key informant or an "insider" who can provide access to others who can help tell the story.

CHAPTER 7

Activity 1
1. a. Scientific; artistic
    b. Naturalistic settings
    c. Day-to-day living
    d. Lived experience
    e. Smaller
    f. Human uniqueness
    g. Research question
2. a. D
    b. A
    c. C
    d. F
    e. B
    f. I
    g. J
    h. G
    i. E
    j. H
3. a. Element 1: Identifying the phenomenon
    1. Study of day-to-day existence for a particular group of individuals
    2. Interested in social processes from perspective of human interactions

      3. Study of the complex cultural aspects related to a phenomenon

      4. An approach for understanding a past event

      5. A focus on an individual, family, a community, an organization, or some other complex phenomenon

b. Element 2: Structuring the study

      1. Query the lived experience, research perspective is bracketed, sample living or has lived the experience

      2. Questions address basic social processes and tend to be action-oriented, researcher brings some knowledge of the literature but exhaustive review is not done prior to beginning the research. The researcher also has concerns about contextual values and that the data are the essence of the theory that emerges. The sample would be participants who have had experience with the circumstances, events, or incidents being studied.

      3. Questions are about lifeways or patterns of behavior within a social context. Researcher attempts to make sense of world from the insider's point of view. The researcher becomes the interpreter of events and tries to make sense and understand them from the emic view. Researchers do this by making their own beliefs explicit and set aside their own biases or assumptions in order to better understand a different world view. The sample often consists of key informants who have knowledge, status, or communication skills about the phenomenon being studied.

      4. Questions are implicit and embedded in the phenomenon studied, researcher understanding of information without imposing interpretation. It is important for the researcher to clearly and carefully identify the event being studied. Data used for the study may be of a primary or secondary nature.

      5. Questions are about issues that serve as a foundation to uncover complexity and pursue understanding. The perspective of the researcher is reflected in the questions. Researchers may choose the most common cases or instead select the most unusual ones.

c. Element 3: Gathering the data

      1. Written or oral data may be collected

      2. Collect data through audiotaped and transcribed interviews and skilled observations

      3. Participant observation, immersion, informant interviews

      4. Use of primary and secondary data sources

      5. Use of interview, observations, document reviews, and other methods

d. Element 4: Analyzing the data

      1. Move from participant's description to researcher synthesis

      2. Data collection and analysis occur simultaneously, use theoretical sampling, constant comparative method, and axial coding

      3. Data are collected and analyzed simultaneously, searching for symbolic categories

      4. Analyze for importance and then validity (authenticity) and reliability

      5. Reflecting and revising meanings

e. Element 5: Describing the findings

      1. A narrative elaboration of the lived experience

      2. Descriptive language to show theory connections to the data

     3. Large quantities of data, provide examples from the data and propositions about relationships of phenomena

     4. Well-synthesized chronicle

     5. A chronologically developed case, a story that describes case dimensions, or vignettes that emphasize various aspects of the case.

4. For example, a personal interest in the health behaviors of families in a culturally unique group of persons might lead to the selection of an ethnographic method to conduct the study. This study method allows the investigator to explore multiple aspects of family life, family households, as well as consider the impact of the situated context on family outcomes. Understanding the health of a specific cultural group may best be understood from the emic and etic perspective gained through observation, interviews, identifying objects used, and determining their value.

Activity 2

1. The main theme of this literature is bone marrow transplantation.

2. A brief history of bone marrow transplantation is provided to inform the reader about some history of the procedure. The authors mention several comprehensive reviews of the literature that were completed in 1994 and 1995.

3. Schuster G, Steeves R, Onega L, and Richardson B (1996). Coping patterns among bone marrow transplant patients: A hermeneutical inquiry, *Cancer Nursing* 19:290–297.

    Steeves R (1992). Patients who have undergone bone marrow transplantation: Their quest for meaning, *Oncol Nurs Forum* 19:899–905.

    These two studies use a qualitative approach to understand the impact of bone marrow transplantation on the recipients. This perspective is far different than thinking about treatment standards or the number of procedures performed. The qualitative studies provide understandings about the patient perspectives as they struggle with their disease and the burdens related to the cure.

4. If they were available, the study authors might have included literature about the impact of participants in bone marrow transplantation from the perspectives of nurses and other health care providers. This addition may help nurses examine their own thoughts and responses to caring for patients having this procedure, which might enable them to examine a topic rarely discussed by colleagues, but pertinent to those involved in care of cancer patients.

Activity 3

1. Hermeneutic phenomenological research

2. Many various web sites might be accessed to gain more insight into hermeneutic phenomenological research. This method tries to explicate or make clear meanings that in some sense are implicit in our action. We know things through our bodies, through our relationships with others, and through our interaction with the things in the environment or world we experience. This is an effective method for inquiring about uniqueness.

3. Five patients who had undergone and survived bone marrow transplants.

4. Patient interviews were conducted privately. Concerns about human subjects such as informed consent and anonymity were addressed. The opening question used with patients was: "What was it like to have a bone marrow transplant?"

5. Interviews were analyzed using the phenomenological approach developed by the Utrecht School of Phenomenology.

Activity 4

1. Twenty patients were interviewed, 15 women and 5 men with a mean age of 46 years.
2. The prevailing theme of the study was the experience of being fearful.
3. Fear of death and hope for survival; fear of the unknown; uncharted physical, mental, and emotional territory; loss of control; and fear of discharge/fear of recurrence.
4. Loss of control, for these patients, meant an inability to control what was occurring in one's life. Loss of control pertained to bodily functions, changes in physical attributes, and emotional losses including personal dignity.

Activity 5

This research could be extremely helpful to nurses and others providing direct care to cancer patients who are being offered bone marrow transplantation as a care option. Careful pre-instructions about what happens before, during, and after the procedure could assist patients to be better prepared for the events and reduce some of the fears they will most likely experience. If nurses can anticipate what patients will feel then they can provide interventions directly linked to these care needs. Information alone may not be enough to prepare the patient, especially the clinical information provided by health professionals. The opportunity to speak with a survivor of the experience may better meet patient's emotional needs.

Activity 6

a. D
b. C
c. B
d. A
e. A
f. B
g. E
h. C
i. D
j. D
k. A
l. C
m. E
n. C
o. D
p. C
q. B
r. A
s. E
t. A (could also be true of B or C)
u. A (could also be B, C, or D)
v. C
w. D (could also be true of A or C)
x. C (could also be A)
y. B
z. C

Activity 7

a. In a dissertation study about family health (Denham, 1997), the method selected to study the phenomenon was ethnography. The researcher wanted to deepen her understanding of the definitions and practices of family health within the household. It required her to operate within the "culture" of that environment.

Other possibilities to consider: *Phenomenology* might be used to investigate the lived experience of family health, *case study* might be used to examine usual cases of family health, and *historical methods* might be used to investigate ways in which family health has changed over the past 100 years.

b. 1. The ways families define health
    2. The ways families use health information
    3. How individuals modify health behaviors
    4. How individuals practice health on a daily basis within the household

c. How do families define and practice family health in their household setting?

d. Families each participated in four audiotaped interviews. Fifteen community informants served as key informants about family health in the community. Participant observation and journal and field notes were also used as data collection methods.

e. Study subjects were located with the assistance of key community informants and snowball techniques. The subjects were eight Appalachian families with preschool children. A total of 39 family members and 15 community informants participated in the study.

f. Data analysis initially involved transcription of the interviews and the use of qualitative computer software to sort and categorize the large quantity of data. The analysis included family cases, but constant comparative methods were used to contrast parents, children, and community informant data.

g. Subjects affirmed the importance of family in producing health, the role of mothers in providing care, the value of early childhood as a time when health behaviors are learned, and the value of the household production of health. Study findings identified that family health was largely a product of family context, family functioning, and family health routines. New knowledge pointed to the complex interactions among family and community that create dynamic and evolving patterns of family health and the identification of family health routines as a way to describe individual and family health behaviors.

As a nurse, the information in this study would encourage me to think about where to focus health teaching. Maybe the best use of resources would be to include health practice education in the pediatrician's office while parents, especially mothers, are waiting with children to see the physician. Maybe we should incorporate health education into Head Start, preschools, and kindergarten. I might also ask more questions about the health practices within a client's family as I try to help the client plan for a change related to health, e.g., ostomy care, diabetic regimen, or an exercise protocol.

CHAPTER 8

Activity 1

The main theme addressed in the data was the topic of patients' fear. Some patients fear dying and only choose bone marrow transplants because no other options exist.

Activity 2

1. Fear in cancer survivors is often related to recurrence of the disease and can be affected by the presence and support of significant others. Nurse-patient communication about these fears needs to be included in assessments and care interventions.
2. Fear and anxiety associated with discharge is a common concern of cancer patients. What kinds of things might nurses do to address these concerns?
3. Loss is described in terms of humiliating acts such as vomiting in front of others and loss of physical control.
4. While cancer patients often experience fears, they are not without hope. This concept has often been identified in many other studies of cancer patients and is supported by the Cohen and Ley (2000) research. In what ways might the nurse clinician use this knowledge about the value of hope to provide better care to cancer patients?
5. This study confirms much of what is already known about the effects of other cancer conditions on patients and provides a more in-depth picture of specifics related to those patients who are having bone marrow transplants as a treatment.
6. Nurse clinicians could easily apply information to ways that they communicate information, provide care, and offer emotional support to cancer patients. What kinds of specific nursing interventions can you identify?

Activity 3

1. a. G
    b. B
    c. D
    d. A
    e. F
    f. D
    g. E
    h. G
    i. B
2. a. Credibility refers to the steps taken in qualitative research to ensure the accuracy, validity, and soundness of the data.
    b. Auditability is a research process that allows the work of a qualitative researcher or a person critiquing a research report to follow the thinking and/or conclusions of a researcher.
    c. Fittingness is the term used to answer these two questions: Are the findings applicable outside the study? Are the results or findings meaningful to persons not involved in the research?

Activity 4

1. When critiquing, it is important to remember that there is not always a single right or wrong answer. It is quite possible to see things from different perspectives and have adequate means of support for your ideas. Therefore, it is quite probable that your classmates may have some answers that are different from yours. It might be helpful to do this activity along with a friend so that you can discuss the different perspectives.
    a. The phenomenon of interest investigated in this report is depression in a group of 12 minority women.
    b. Better understandings are needed about minority groups and cultural differences that result in some groups being at higher risk than others. Depression is a form

of mental illness that is widespread, but many experience a stigma associated with having the disease and may be slow in seeking treatment or may not seek any formal care. A study of this problem is of concern to nursing.

c,e. The researchers provide an ample description of their research methods and these techniques are appropriate for grounded theory methodology and are compatible with the subject being investigated.

d. While the sample size is small, it is similar to what is observed in other studies using grounded theory. The authors fail to tell the reader exactly how the participants were recruited. The subjects are described based upon culture and location of birth, but we know nothing about their age or socioeconomic status. The participants were relatively well-educated and this leads to questioning whether less-educated women would have explained a similar experience.

f. The researchers carefully describe the strategies used to analyze the data. However, a new student of research may not clearly understand what is implied by "open coding, categorizing, linking, expansion, and reduction until hypotheses were generated" (p. 40).

g,h,i. The topics of credibility, auditability, and fittingness of the data are not made explicit in the research report. However, the fact that they are not directly discussed within the article might be a matter of page limits for publication rather than good or bad science on the part of the researchers.

j. The study findings are clearly presented and the reader is able to understand the participants' experience and the theoretical perspective. The process of "being strong" was what these minority women described as how they coped with the social stigma of depression, personal relationships, and belief in Christian doctrine. "Being strong" was described as four sub-processes: "dwelling on it," "diverting myself," "regaining my composure," and "trying new approaches." The authors carefully describe each of these phenomena. While there are a number of direct quotes from participants included, the reader relies heavily upon the expertise of the researchers for the assurance that these conceptualizations are true to the data. In the section entitled "Diverting Myself: Beginning to Manage," the authors use a number of references from other published literature to demonstrate that the authors are placing these findings within the context of what is already known.

The conclusions provide a nice summary for the reader and state that the study adds to the understandings about valuing cultural and social contexts where women construct their lives. The authors strongly address the issues of cultural sensitivity and culturally competent care, areas of concern to nursing practice. They identify several relevant questions for future research including the possibility that "being strong" could induce depression and slow and/or prevent recovery for some women.

2. Given a chance to speak with the researchers, two questions that might be asked are: What in your background caused you to be interested in studying depression in this population? You imply that in some cases "being strong" might be a more negative than positive attribute, could you discuss this more fully?

Activity 5
Your teacher may want to send you to some specific Internet links for additional learning about various aspects of qualitative research.

CHAPTER 9

Activity 1
1. d
2. c
3. e
4. g
5. h
6. f
7. b
8. a

Activity 2
1. Maturation. The mothers' confidence could be increased by any number of factors, including the act of caring for their infant during the month. The time of measurement could be immediately prior to discharge. Use of a control group would strengthen the findings.
2. Instrumentation. The use of standardized calibrated equipment and training for the volunteers would increase the internal validity of the findings.
3. History. The increase in taxes could account for a decrease in the rate of cigarette smoking. Use of a control group and randomization would improve interpretation of the findings.
4. Selection bias. The differences in smoking cessation rates could be attributed to a number of motivational factors. Random assignment to smoking cessation groups is needed to strengthen this design.
5. Mortality. The program is not successful for single homeless women with preschool children. It is important to look at the make-up of the final study sample when the results are interpreted.
6. Testing. Taking the test repeatedly may be the factor leading to an increase in confidence and accuracy, rather than the experimental program. The use of different outcome instruments and measures may be necessary.

Activity 3
1. The setting consisted of "Cardiac units in two large community hospitals (between 400- and 500-bed facilities) located in a Midwest metropolitan area with a population of 2 million. . ." If we thought it necessary or were just curious we might speculate that the metropolitan area was Minneapolis, Minnesota since two of the three researchers were associated with the University of Minneapolis *and* Minneapolis would be designated as "Midwest" while Baltimore would not.
2. The subjects were 180 elder/caregiver dyads. Remember that while the dyads were the unit of analysis there were 360 individuals involved.
3. The investigators outlined five criteria that were used to select the participants. The criteria were used to select the elders who would be invited to participate. The criteria included the requirement of an identified caregiver who would participate. The five criteria are outlined in the second column of page 448 in the text. See the first paragraph under the heading of "Sample."

    You would also consider the selection of the hospitals to be used in the study. The investigators tell you that the hospitals were "matched in terms of size, type, and discharge-planning practices used in cardiac units" (page 448 of text, column 1, under

"Design"). Random selection was used to determine which hospital would receive the treatment and which would serve as control.

4. No major area of information is missing. I found the description of the design, setting, and sample very clear. I would have liked to know the span of time from the first interview with the first subject to the final 2 months postdischarge interview with the last subject.

   My curiosity was piqued with the mention of the CHF critical pathway in Hospital 1. I wondered if there were some fundamental differences in the administration and staff of the hospitals that led to the change in Hospital 1 which led me to think about how difficult matching of samples/subjects can be. My curiosity would not be something I would have expected the investigators to answer in the research report, but it is something I might ask about if our paths crossed at a meeting.

5. Yes, the sample was homogeneous. There was no reason to suspect that there were any extraneous variables that systematically affected one group and not the other.

   This is the area that *could* make the length of time the study required from beginning to end important. If something had happened to the area around one hospital but not the other, e.g. a tornado or a fire, the event could have systematically changed the data provided by those subjects. We have to trust that the investigators would have informed us if such an event had occurred. Think about all of the research studies that may have been affected by the events of September 11, 2001.

6. The variables were measured using the Discharge Planning Questionnaire to identify the initial need for follow-up care. In-person interviews and telephone interviews of elders and caregivers were conducted at the designated time intervals. The instruments used to collect data were described in table format (Table 2 on page 450).

   I would have liked a bit more information regarding the actual conduct of the interviews. The "research team" is mentioned in page 449 (top of column 2) but there is no information provided about how consistency across interviews was maintained. There had to be more than one interviewer (given there were approximately 900 interviews conducted), and we have no information about how the interviews were constructed nor how individual differences in interview style was handled. A couple of sentences would have handled this concern. Please keep in mind that the information may have been in the original report but was deleted for editorial reasons.

7. Hospital 1 served as the control group.

Activity 4

1. Yes. The investigators were interested in the outcomes associated with a new type of discharge planning. They compared the "new" with the "old" or the currently used standard method of discharge planning. A question of this type requires testing the new against the old in the same time frame. The chosen design allowed the investigators to do this.

2. Yes. Collection of information about the subjects before any intervention occurred and collection of information from a comparison group that did not receive the intervention allowed the investigators to be more confident that their findings were the result of the intervention. This design (nonequivalent control group) differs from the true experimental design only in the lack of random assignment of subjects to either the control or intervention group which would have been impractical.

3. No, this study is beyond the expectations for either a master's thesis or a doctoral dissertation. The complexity of the study, the length of time involved in the data collec-

tion, and the overall cost of the study would create impractical hurdles for the typical graduate student.

4. Yes, the parts of the study fit together. The initial clinical concern is supported by the literature which links directly to the hypotheses and leads to chosen design.

5. Common threats to internal validity in the nonequivalent control group design are selection, maturation, testing, and mortality. The threats of history and instrumentation are of no more concern with this design than any other. Specific considerations would be:

Selection:	Bull, Hansen, and Gross (2000) (Appendix A of text) established criteria for selection of subjects and had an experimental and control site.
Maturation:	Maturation of the elders would be expected to be minimal since they were adults in the same age range and were assessed initially using a measure of cognitive competence. It was unclear from the report as to how maturation may have affected the caregiver group.
Testing:	The number of instruments used, their variety, and the length of time between testing periods could have minimized the effects of repeated testing. The concern with repeated testing is that subjects will remember how they responded the last time and that this memory will influence their response this time. However, the number and variety of instruments used in this study would make it difficult to remember responses from one interview time to another. There may have been a testing affect *because* of the number of instruments, and it is unclear about the type of control used in this area. The fatigue factor could influence the response to those instruments used at the end of each interview. If the same instrument was given last in every instance the scores on that instrument may reflect "real" change or may reflect fatigue.
Mortality:	The investigators explained the loss of subjects from the beginning of the study to the end of the study. See page 448, column 2, bottom of first paragraph under "Sample."
History:	Unanticipated daily events did influence this study. The implementation of the CHF critical pathway in one hospital confounded the outcomes. It would have been impossible for the investigators to determine which outcomes were related to which discharge planning protocol.
Instrumentation:	There is no reason to think that the instruments changed during the course of the study.

6. Selection effects, reactive effects, and measurement effects are the three major threats to external validity.

Selection:	The investigators caution the reader when they point out that the subjects in this study were predominantly Anglo which limits generalization. They also encourage thinking about the influence of culture on the acceptability of the proposed intervention.
Reactive:	It is possible that there could have been some positive outcomes simply from being included in the study, i.e. individuals paid more attention to care and/or wanted to help the researchers. Controlling for this effect, e.g. adding a third group that was given the same amount of attention but not the specific intervention, would have added considerable cost.

Measurement: It is possible that the pretesting created a focus in the intervention group that was not present in the control group. The investigators had a built-in control for this possibility (testing individuals in one hospital without use of the intervention), but this was the hospital that changed its discharge planning procedure and the data had to be eliminated.

CHAPTER 10

Activity 1
1. Solomon four-group
2. Time series
3. After-only experiment
4. After-only nonequivalent control group
5. True experiment
6. Nonequivalent control group

Activity 2
1. Before-and-after nonequivalent control group design
2. Quasiexperimental because subjects were not randomly assigned to the treatment/intervention or control groups. Random assignment of one hospital to serve as the control (which left the second hospital as the treatment site) provided some control over possible investigator bias but could do nothing about variables that *could* have been operating in the two different groups of people. There *may* be some systematic difference between the individuals who would go to hospital A and those who would go to hospital B. Random assignment of the hospitals to either treatment or control group would not address these variables.
3. The antecedent variable would be "a" (difference in caregivers).
   The intervening variable would be "b" (new CHF critical pathway).
4. The major implication would be that the type of discharge planning can make a difference. The potential exists to benefit clients (increased sense of continuity of care) and organizations (reduction in cost). Additional work needs to be done before a specific form of discharge planning can be recommended.

Activity 3
1.

	Pretest	Teaching	Post-Test
Group A	X	X	X
Group B		X	X
Group C	X		X
Group D			X

(*Note:* The groups may be arranged in any order, but the four group pattern must be followed.)
2. The nurses would be randomly assigned to each of the groups using a table of random numbers or computer random assignment.
3. The pain knowledge and attitudes questionnaire would be used as a pretest.
4. The teaching program is the experimental treatment.

5. The pain knowledge and attitudes questionnaire is also the post-test or outcome measure.
6. The Solomon four-group design is ideal for experimental studies in which the pretest might affect the outcome. In this case, the questionnaire might change nurses' knowledge and attitudes about pain management. The researcher will be able to compare results for nurses receiving the teaching and not receiving the teaching with and without the pretest.
7. This type of design is particularly effective in ruling out threats to internal validity that the before-and-after groups may experience. It is effective for highly sensitive issues that might be affected by simply completing a questionnaire as a baseline pretest.
8. A disadvantage of the Solomon four-group design is that a large number of subjects must be available for assignment into the four groups.

Activity 4

1. a. Quasiexperimental, nonequivalent control group design
    b. The presence of a pretest allows the investigator to compare the two groups on important antecedent variables before the intervention (treatment variable) is implemented.
    c. Minimal confidence that the intervention (treatment) group and the comparison (control) group were similar at the beginning of the study.
2. a. Quasiexperimental; interrupted time series design with a nonequivalent control group. If you indicated: (i) it was some type of a time series design and (ii) the comparison group could not be considered to be equivalent to the treatment group because of the different data collection periods and methods, you have captured the essence of the design.
    b. To quote the investigators: "Anecdotal evidence of the positive effects of the TTM [the thermal mattress] on the body temperatures of VLBW [very-lo- birth-weight] infants made it unethical to withhold its use; therefore, randomization was not possible." (L'Herault, Petroff, & Jeffrey, 2001, p. 212)
3. a. Time series design
    b. The advantage of this type of design is that though it is not possible to use random assignment, the uses of a group similar in characteristics other than irritability allow the researcher to make comparisons. In longitudinal studies, each subject can be compared with himself over time to allow trends to be observed.
    c. The disadvantage of this quasiexperimental design is that cause and effect relationships are more difficult to determine when random assignment is not made. The researcher has to carefully examine and compare the groups to determine whether another factor accounts for the differences observed.

Activity 5

1. Quasiexperimental designs are usually more practical, more feasible, and more adaptable to real-world practice. In many studies important to nursing, it is not possible to randomize subjects into groups for practical or ethical reasons.
2. The researcher must carefully examine other factors that could account for differences between groups.
3. The clinician must carefully critique the research study and also look for other factors that might explain the results of the study. The results of any study with any design must be evaluated to determine if other factors influence the findings. The results should also be compared with the findings of other similar studies.

Activity 6

The author found 953,000 at the time of manuscript submission.

The website is based at Tuskegee University and is "devoted to engaging the sciences, humanities, law and religious faiths in the exploration of the core moral issues which underlie research and medical treatment of African-American and other underserved people."

CHAPTER 11

Activity 1

1. Survey
2. Longitudinal
3. Correlational
4. Ex post facto
5. Cross-sectional
6. Correlational
7. Cross-sectional
8. Survey
9. Cross-sectional
10. Cross-sectional

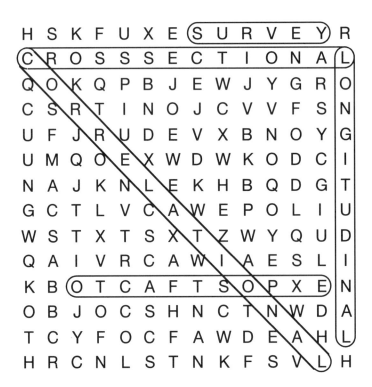

Activity 2

	Advantages	Disadvantages
Correlation studies	A3	D1, D3, D4, D7
Cross-sectional	A1	D2, D5
Ex post facto	A4	D1, D2, D3, D4, D5, D7
Longitudinal	A2, A6	D2, D8
Prospective	A2, A7	D3, D4, D7, D8
Retrospective	A4	D1, D2, D3, D4, D5, D7
Survey	A1	D5, D7

Activity 3

1, SC, L Comparative, longitudinal would be the best fit. The term "longitudinal" most often is used when investigators collect data from a group three or more times. Data were collected in this study only twice but there was a span of time between the two measures, and the investigators were describing change over time.
2. SD or SE (descriptive or exploratory)
3. CS (cross-sectional)
4. SD (descriptive)
5. LS (longitudinal, survey)
6. M (methodological)

Activity 4

1. Design-descriptive, exploratory
2. Yes, one of the major points of the text's authors was that consumers must be wary of nonexperimental studies that make causal claims about the findings unless a causal modeling technique is used. No such model was used in the Mohr study. It appears that the author may have attempted to show a cause-and-effect relationship among the variables that is not appropriate for an exploratory, nonexperimental study.

Activity 5

Ex post facto

CHAPTER 12

Activity 1

1. P
2. N
3. P
4. N
5. N
6. P
7. P

Activity 2

1. b
2. f

3. d
4. a
5. c
6. e

Activity 3
1. a. Yes, overall, the sample was adequately described. A reader can picture the group that completed the questionnaires and since this was an exploratory study complicated demographic information was unnecessary. It would have been helpful to know the total enrollment of the middle school and the distribution of the total enrollment on the variables mentioned, e.g. gender and ethnicity. Having this information would have allowed the reader to form an opinion about how well the group represented the school population.
    b. Maybe if the population were defined as students in this particular middle school, but we weren't given that information. The sample would not be representative of all seventh and eighth graders.
    c. Nonprobability sample
    d. Yes, given the exploratory nature of the study the sample size was adequate.
2. Easier to obtain subjects because the investigators use those who volunteer.
3. The disadvantages of convenience samples include increased risk of inherent bias, and increased risk of the sample not representing the population.

Activity 4
1. True
2. True
3. False
4. False
5. True
6. True

Activity 5
1. Yes, the characteristics of the sample were well described.
2. Yes. The population inferred for this study would be all adolescents (people between the age of 12 and 21 years) in the 134 schools sampled. Given that the students were part of a national study one could infer that the investigators were interested in all U.S. adolescents.
3. Yes, for the most part. The investigators rely on the reader's being familiar with the characteristics of the U.S. adolescent population. You will be able to make this determination after you have reviewed the two web sites listed in the study guide.
4. Criteria for sample eligibility were not specified. The description of the procedure noted the use of a systematic random sampling strategy and referred the reader to a separate article for a more detailed explanation. It was not clear how the 134 schools were selected nor what percentage of U.S. secondary schools is represented by these 134 schools. Again, this may be explained in the other article.
5. Based on the material provided to you in this study guide you would have to answer "no." In fact, delimitations were discussed later in the article.
6. Yes, it would be possible to replicate the study sample. It would be expensive and time-consuming to do so and probably not practical, but it could be done.

7. Again, we are referred to the 1997 article that is devoted to the research design used in for the national longitudinal study.
8. The most frequently cited source of bias would the missing of an important variable that would influence the findings. For example, if the investigators stratified the sample based on five variables while unknown to them there was a sixth variable that was very influential.
9. The sample size is appropriate. It is not substantiated in the excerpt that you read.
10. Yes, as described in the excerpt ". . .all respondents provided informed consent." (p. 23).
11. Yes, the investigators discussed the limitations of generalizing the findings.
12. Yes, the investigators discuss areas that would benefit from further research.

CHAPTER 13

Activity 1
1. Nursing research committee
2. Justice
3. Expedited review
4. Unethical research study
5. Institutional review board

Activity 2
1. Respect for persons
2. Beneficence
3. Justice

Activity 3
1. Bull, Hansen, and Gross obtained the approval of the institutional review boards at both universities and both hospitals for the study. They sought the permission of the charge nurse on the cardiac units before approaching elders who met the criteria. Permission was obtained from each elder and from each caregiver.
2. Cohen and Ley asked subjects to participate and interviewed only those who consented. They mention that the subjects signed informed consent documents which would lead one to think that the study had been approved by the hospital's institutional review board but such approval is not explicitly stated. The investigators specifically mention the need to protect the clients'/subjects' anonymity and did so by changing identifying information and using an interviewer who was not a member of the unit's staff.
3. Mahon, Yarcheski, and Yarcheski had their study approved by the university's institutional review board. The principal and the teachers at the selected middle school approved the instrument packets. All students were provided with an information packet. Students who chose to participate and who had their parents' consent completed the data collection instruments.
4. LoBiondo-Wood, Williams, Kouzekanani, and McGhee received approval from an institutional review board. It is not clear whether this was the university's or the hospital's IRB or a joint university/medical center IRB. The subjects were contacted by mail and returned the consent form and completed instruments in person or by return mail.

Activity 4

1. (a-d) Children, elderly, mentally ill, the unborn, persons with AIDS, people in institutions, vulnerable populations (e.g., students or prisoners)
2. a. Bull, Hansen, and Gross worked with the elderly who are identified as a vulnerable population.
   b. Cohen and Ley worked with clients who had undergone bone marrow transplants. These individuals are not designated as a vulnerable population but are considered to be an "oversubscribed research population" and require special attention.
   c. Mahon, Yarcheski, and Yarcheski collected data from children between the ages of 12–14. They are considered to be a vulnerable population.
   d. LoBiondo-Wood, Williams, Kouzekanani, and McGhee collected data from the mothers of children who were being evaluated for a liver transplant. They are not considered a vulnerable population.
3. a. The subjects in this study are students. They are a vulnerable population, and therefore, extra precautions must be undertaken to protect their rights.
   b. The subjects in this study were adolescents, who make up a vulnerable population, and prisoners, who are both a captive and convenient population, thus extra precautions would need to be taken to guard their rights.

Activity 5

Note: Each student's answer will be different. However, at San Jose State University the composition of the Institutional Review Board: Human Subjects is as follows: one seat designated for a nursing representative, another for a psychology faculty member, a member from Graduate Studies & Research, two student health representatives, a biology representative, a College of Education representative, a Faculty-at-Large member, a Community-at-Large representative, and a student representative. It is informative to note that the programs that have graduate students doing a large number of studies with human subjects such as nursing and psychology have designated seats; also of note is that it is not composed exclusively of faculty but that there is one student and one community member.

Activity 6

(Answers will vary)

1. I had not really thought about this before. I have difficulty with this question because I teach a research course with 75 to 90 students each semester and encourage them to think of research questions continually; and I would not expect to be acknowledged if a classroom discussion led to a thesis. I believe an acknowledgment would be necessary if the faculty member or clinical mentor spent individual time helping someone to refine a research question or problem.
2. I do not believe so. I am compulsive, as most nurses are, about documentation.
3. Again, this is problematic because of the amount of time and energy that might go into duplicating the material. Although ethically I would feel obligated to share the data, I also believe it would be appropriate to ask for funding for duplicating and any other expenses incurred.

Activity 7

1. One ethical principle guiding research is beneficence; this imparts an obligation to do no harm and maximize possible benefits. Therefore, it would not be ethical to conduct an

experimental study at this time. Instead, I would do a descriptive or qualitative study describing the patients and their symptoms and the treatments being used, and then begin to identify all the variables involved.

2. The population of interest is children, who are one of the vulnerable groups; extra precautions must be undertaken to protect their rights. However, at that time there were no guidelines identifying children as a vulnerable population; nor was the Nuremberg Code, which was the original code of ethics for research that was developed after World War II, yet developed. In research involving children, parental consent is required.

3. The study would have to be descriptive, or qualitative, describing in detail all the variables involved.

Activity 8

Web site originates in Canada

Moloney states that recognition as a profession requires: (a) more autonomy, (b) higher sense of commitment, and (c) standardized education.

CHAPTER 14

Activity 1

Study 1

1. c. In-person and telephone interviews

2. The investigators interviewed each member of the dyads in nine areas. It is possible that interviewing provided a consistent way to collect the information without worrying about the subjects' reading ability, eyesight acuity, or skill and coordination in writing. The investigators do not specify why they chose this particular method.

Study 2

1. c. Open-ended interviews

2. The investigators wanted to understand the patients' (subjects') experience with an autologous bone marrow transplantation. This was an initial study and the investigators wanted to hear everything the subjects wanted to share. They did not have any preconceived ideas about what areas or variables would be important, so they chose not to impose a structure on the data collection.

3. In my opinion it was a successful data collection method. The data they obtained is very rich and points to areas that need further study so RNs can improve their care of clients experiencing this procedure.

Study 3

1. d. Questionnaire

2. Questionnaires were the choice in this study because the investigators had definite questions they wanted answered, they were collecting data from a large group of people at the same time, and the individuals could remain anonymous.

Study 4

1. d. Questionnaire

2. The education level of the mothers (20 of the 29) had attended or graduated from college. The reading level would be sufficient to complete seven instruments, of which six were standardized instruments.

Activity 2
1. Consumers
2. Physiological
3. Reactivity
4. Interviews
5. Records
6. Questionnaires
7. Objectivity, consistency
8. Concealment
9. Interrater reliability
10. Operationalization
11. Likert scale
12. Content analysis
13. Fun

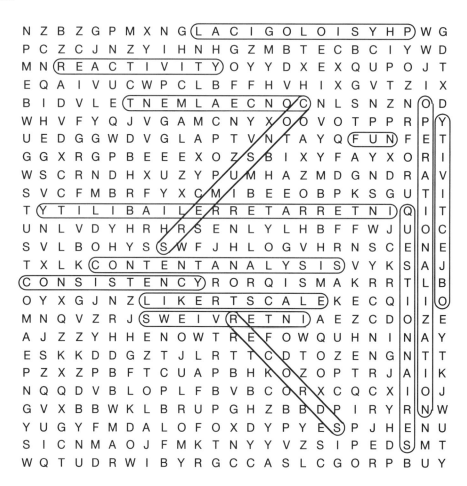

Activity 3
1. Children; interactions between people when the investigator is not part of the interaction; psychiatric patients; classrooms

2. The consent is usually of the type where permission to observe for a specified purpose is requested. The specific behaviors that are to be observed are not named. The use of the data and degree of anonymity are explained. In some situations, the subjects will be asked to review the data after the observation and before inclusion in the data pool.
3. Reactivity is the major concern when the investigator has reason to believe that his/her presence will change the nature of the subjects' behavior.

Activity 4

Physiological measures would be of minimal use since the data I am seeking would not involve actual measures of the residents' physiological status. Not particularly interested in current blood pressure, temperature, urinary output, etc.

Could consider using observation, e.g. sitting in an emergency room and observing the types of health care concerns that enter. Would need to think about whether this would be observation with concealment. Would need to wrestle with the notion of what is private information and what is public domain information.

Could use questionnaires and collect data from all types of health care providers. Could give me a lot of data in a short time. Wonder how busy they would be and what would be the probability of their filling out the questionnaire?

Could use an interview. Is costly in terms of researcher time, but could get me the information in more detail because I could ask them to expand upon specific items. But who would I want to interview? How do I get into their offices/homes, etc.?

Need to get some information from the people who actually live here. Wonder how I could reach a cross-section of those individuals? Could I call? What about those people without a telephone?

Better check out the census data to get a clearer picture of what I am dealing with. Probably have some morbidity and mortality data collected by the state health department. I would probably utilize existing records to get a first sense of what the parameters of "health" are in this community. Then I would talk to some people about who knew the most about this area and arrange some interviews with these individuals. These would be guided interviews with open-ended items to encourage the sharing of as much information as possible. I would also seek a way to collect data from a variety of health care users, e.g. surveys in the waiting room of various agencies, maybe the crowd at a mall, at a county fair.

One data collection instrument would not be sufficient to collect the information needed about the areas addressed.

Activity 5

1. d
2. a
3. d
4. a, b, c
5. d

Activity 6

1. NDNQI = National Database of Nursing Quality Indicators
2. Ten quality indicators form the core.
3. Form would be categorized as a survey.

CHAPTER 15

Activity 1
1. S; avoided by proper calibration of the scale.
2. S; decrease error by providing instructions, ensuring confidentiality, or other means to allow students to freely express themselves.
3. R; lessen by training research assistants and using strict protocols or rule books to guide analysis.
4. R; decrease their anxiety by addressing their concerns, providing comfort measures or other efforts that might decrease their anxiety. Anxiety may alter the test responses.

Activity 2
1. Construct validity
2. Face validity
3. Content validity
4. Construct validity
5. Construct validity or convergent validity
6. Convergent validity; contrasted groups; divergent validity; factor analysis; hypothesis testing
7. Concurrent validity; criterion validity

Activity 3
1. Stability; homogeneity; equivalence
2. Test-retest methods could be accomplished by giving the same test again at a later date and seeing if the two scores are highly correlated. Parallel or alternate forms, such as alternate versions of the same test, could also be used to establish stability.
3. Alternate forms would be better if the test taker is likely to remember and be influenced by the items or the answers from the first test.
4. a. 2
   b. 4
   c. 1
   d. 3
5. a. Yes
   b. Cronbach's alpha for each instrument in previous studies and in the current one.
   c. The information provided would increase my confidence in the results of this study.

Activity 4
Current smoker, B/P screening, height, weight, BMI, and several demographic variables

Activity 5
1. Six instruments
2. See the completed table and remarks.

Critiquing Questions

Instrument	#1	#2	#3	#4	#5	#6	#7
State Anger	Y	Y	Y	Y	n/a	Y	Y
Trait Anger	Y	Y	Y	Y	n/a	Y	Y
AGWB	Y	Y	Y	Y	n/a	N*	N*
Symptom Pattern	Y	Y	Y	Y	n/a	N*	N*
Vigor-Activity	Y	Y	Y	Y	n/a	N*	N*
Change Subscale	Y	Mixed	Y	Y	n/a	N*	Y

*Strengths and weaknesses were not explicitly discussed in this report. Good evidence was provided by the test statistics reported in the article, but specific limitations of each instrument (either in general or specifically related to this study) were not discussed. This information could have been included in the original draft of the study but easily could have been eliminated by the editors for space reasons.

The reliability statistics on the Change Subscale were not consistently at the minimally expected level of .70. When the subscale was used in an earlier study with adolescents the reliability data had not been reported. One reliability report on its use with college students was in the accepted range but the other was not. The KR-20 for the sample in this study was .68 which, while close to .70, did not reach that desired correlation. Taking all of this together the discussion section appropriately considered the instrument as needing a closer look in future studies.

CHAPTER 16

Activity 1
1. d
2. c
3. d
4. a
5. a, b, or c
6. a
7. b
8. d
9. a
10. c

Activity 2
1. a. Pain. Pain is the only variable identified in this excerpt. We do not know whether it is being used as an independent or dependent variable. It is most often identified as a dependent variable.

    b.   Level of measurement is ordinal.
2. a.   Independent variables are race, types of MI symptoms.
    b.   Dependent variable is prehospital delay time.
    c.   Level of measurement of each variable
       Race = nominal
       Types of MI symptoms = nominal
       Prehospital delay time = interval or ratio
3. a.   Independent variable is psychoeducational intervention
    b.   Dependent variables are emotional health, functional health status, satisfaction.
    c.   Level of measurement of each variable
       Intervention = nominal. A subject experienced the intervention or a subject did not experience the intervention.
       Emotional health = ordinal. Subjects were asked to report *frequency* data which will allow the investigators to count how many times each symptom was marked and be able to rank subjects according to the frequency of symptoms.
       Functional health status = ordinal in the most conservative use of data but might be treated as interval data if the instrument has been so constructed. You would need to review the instrument.
       Satisfaction = ordinal. Subjects *rated* various areas. Ratings usually imply the use of some type of scale, e.g. on a scale of 1 to 5 or 1 to 7 or 1 to 10. The same comment about whether these would be measurements at the ordinal level or the interval level applies. Remember for a scale to be truly interval the investigator needs to be able to assure the reader that the distance between intervals is equal.
4. a.   Variable being measured is anxiety.
    b.   Level of measurement is ratio. All three of these measures would be regarded as ratio.

Activity 3
1. a.   Clinical symptoms of MI
    b.   Percentage of each symptom based on frequency of each symptom in each of the two groups of subjects
    c.   Nominal
    d.   Yes
    e.   Yes
2. a.   Variables are sedation or medications and duration of procedure.
    b.   Level of measurement: Technically ratio would fit both variables. I say *technically* because time is a funny variable. In a theoretical sense there can be a position of no time, but in a practical sense, zero time is not helpful.
    c.   Yes
    d.   Descriptive data: dosage column and standard deviation (SD) column which also is related to the dosage numbers.
    e.   SD is a measure of variation. The larger the standard deviation the more heterogeneous the sample.

Activity 4

Across
1. j Goofy's best friend
3. e Old abbreviation for mean
5. b Abbreviation for number of measures in a given data set (the measures may be individual people or some smaller piece of data like blood pressure readings)
8. m Describes a set of data with a standard deviation of 3 when compared with a set of data with a standard deviation of 12
10. h Abbreviation for standard deviation
11. f Marks the "score" where 50% of the scores are higher and 50% are lower
12. c Measure of variation that shows the lowest and highest number in a data set

Down
1. l The values that occur most frequently in a data set
2. i 68% of the values in a normal distribution fall between ±1 of this statistic
4. d Can describe the height of a distribution
6. g Describes a distribution characterized by a tail
7. k Very unstable
9. a Measure of central tendency used with interval of ratio data

Activity 5
1. 91%
2. Rural setting of school and junior high; rural setting of school and senior high
3. Elementary grade
4. Yes, table and text agree.

Activity 6
1. a. The questions asked were about "differences" which means there is a comparison of data from two or more groups. The bulk of the analysis would rely on inferential statistics. Some descriptive statistics may be anticipated in the analysis of demographic data.
   b. This is a qualitative study; therefore, one would expect little use of statistics. Again, descriptive strategies may be used to describe the study's subjects.
   c. Again, the investigators in this study were interested in comparisons between data. Descriptive strategies would play a small part in the analysis.
   d. The study is described as being exploratory which would lead the reader to think that the bulk of the analysis would be descriptive, and it is. Correlations are used, and it is easy to think inferential statistics are being used when levels of statistical significance are mentioned. In this particular case correlations are used to better describe the relationship between variables.
2. a. Yes, see p. 451 for the description of readmissions and trips to the ER.
   b. Yes, see description of subjects on p. 459.
   c. Yes, see description of the sample on p. 473 in the section head "Procedure."
   d. Yes, see description of the sample on pp. 481, 482 and the way the correlations are discussed in the results section.
3. a. Yes, see p. 451 for the description of readmissions and trips to the ER.
   b. Yes, see description of subjects on p. 459

  c. Yes, see description of the sample on p. 473.
  d. Yes, see description of the sample on pp. 481, 482 and the way the correlations are discussed in the results section.
4. Yes, descriptive statistics were used appropriately in all of the studies.
5. The LoBiondo-Wood, Williams, Kouzekanani, & McGhee studied utilized descriptive statistics to the greatest extent.

Activity 7
Body 23–32″ long; tail 12–20″; 11-30 lbs.

CHAPTER 17

Activity 1
Remember that each person's set of cards will contain the essential information about each inferential tool. You can keep these cards with your study materials and pull out the appropriate card as you read a study that uses the statistic. It won't be long before you can read the inferential statistics portion of a study without using the cards.

Activity 2
1. Null hypothesis
2. ANOVA, parametric statistics
3. Research hypothesis
4. Sampling error
5. Parameter, sample
6. Correlation
7. Type II, Type I
8. Probability
9. Practical significance
10. Nonparametric statistics
11. Statistical significance
12. Research hypothesis, null hypothesis
13. c; b; a; e; d

Activity 3
1. The basic question addressed by Bull, Hansen and Gross was to examine the differences in outcomes for elders and caregivers and costs associated with two types of hospital discharge planning.
2. The hypotheses were stated. There were eight in total. Four were written out and a blanket statement, "The same hypotheses were posited for 2 months postdischarge," covered the other four hypotheses.
3. Scores on perceived health will be the same (*or* no different *or* will show no differences) for clients in the intervention and control cohorts.
4. Allows the investigators to test whether the stated relationship is different from zero.

5. Independent variables:
      1. Standard discharge planning protocol
      2. Partnership model of discharge planning

   Dependent variables:
      1. Perceived health
      2. Satisfaction
      3. Caregivers' response
      4. Resource use

6. Addresses "differences between/among groups"
7. Two
8. There were several measures taken for each of the dependent variables. For example, perceived health used data from the Short Form-36 and the Symptom Questionnaire. Table 3 of the report lists the scores for the elder clients across all instruments. The table also contains the information as to which scores were expressed in means (interval or ratio level of measurement) and which scores were expressed as a median (ordinal level of measurement).
9. a. Two groups, looking for differences, and interval data = use the t-statistic
   b. Two groups, looking for differences, and ordinal data = Mann Whitney U statistic
10. Yes
11. I would prefer the partnership model of discharge planning. I would anticipate having more information, less negative reaction to being the caregiver, and feeling better.
12. (Please note that I am treating this finding as one of the hypotheses when it was not explicitly stated as one.)

   The results indicated that there was a statistically significant difference between the caregivers in the partnership model of discharge and those in the standard discharge protocol with the partnership model caregivers feeling better at 2 weeks and 2 months postdischarge. The null hypothesis would be that there would be NO differences between the two groups.

   A Type I error would be that the null hypothesis was in fact true. The investigators found a difference for some reason (usually connected to the setting of the level of probability associated with the particular statistic used) when there really was not a difference between the groups. In this situation the interpretation would be that both groups of caregivers reported the same level of health status.

   In this particular study there would be very few, if any, practical concerns with the finding of "no difference" between the groups.

Activity 4

1. a. Inferential statistics were t-statistic and chi-square.
   b. t-statistic for age because the data are interval/ratio; chi-square for the variables of ethnicity, health conditions, smoking, exercise, and immunizations because these data are nominal
   c. Groups were regular patient and episodic patient.
2. a. Inferential statistic: F, ANOVA
   b. Because there were repeated measures of anxiety; four measures of state anxiety for each person
3. a. Two groups
   b. The groups differed in that one received tap water enema and the other received soapsuds enema
   c. There was no statistical significance in the average amount of enema solution given to the subjects in each group. OR The difference in the average amount of solution

given to those in each group could have happened by chance, the difference wasn't big enough to think there were any systematic differences between the groups.)

d. The information provided is that there was a big enough difference between the amount of return (net output) following the enema that something other than chance was operating. Given the design of the study one would be led to think that the difference was due to the type of enema administered. You would need to read the complete study before you came to any definite conclusions.

The use of the *t*-statistic was appropriate because the comparison was between the means of two groups (tap water and soapsuds) and the data were measured using a ratio scale (grams of output following an enema).

Activity 5

There are 10 leading health indicators.

The three reasons are: (a) ability to motivate others, (b) availability of data to measure, and (c) importance as a public health issue.

". . . samples design uses State-level, random-digit-dialed probability sample of the adult (aged 18 years and over) population."

CHAPTER 18

Activity 1

1. a. A
    b. B
    c. B
    d. B
    e. A
    f. A
    g. A
    h. B
    i. B
    j. B

Activity 2

1. a. Yes for the most part. The information **supplements that found in the text**, which allows the **text to be economical** in the presentation of the findings. It condenses data that would be very confusing and would require several paragraphs if explained in the narrative style found in text. **The title is precise**. It would be possible to interpret data from this table alone. A reader would not need the text to be able to pull relevant information from Table 2. It does **repeat the text** in the sense that the data highlighted in the text appear in the table, but the table is not limited to the information found in the text. The table contains a lot of data which can intimidate a reader, but given the richness of the data in this study it could be misleading to the reader to condense the data in the table much more.
    b. Most likely to be using cocaine were students who used all three types of tobacco.
    c. Alcohol was the substance reported most used and those who "smoked cigarettes only" used it the most of all the groups.

Activity 3

Obviously I cannot provide you with "the answer" to this item. The intent of including such an exercise is to give you a taste of what goes into designing a table. As the variables increase in number and complexity and the sheer quantity of the data expands, it becomes more and more difficult to create concise but helpful tables.

Activity 4

1. a.   "N = 141" means the sample consisted of 141 subjects.
    b.   Well-being
    c.   Standard deviation (SD) is the largest at 29.80 and the range is 47-193.
2. a.   1.   Trait and state anger
         2.   Vigor and state anger
         3.   Vigor and trait anger
         4.   Change and trait anger
         5.   Change and state anger
         6.   Symptom patterns and state anger
         7.   Symptom patterns and trait anger
         8.   Well-being and state anger
         9.   Well-being and trait anger
    b.   The relationship between trait anger and symptom patterns is positive meaning that as the subjects' level of trait anger increased so did the reported symptom patterns. The reverse is true for trait anger and well-being. This is a negative relationship. As trait anger increases the subjects' report of well-being decreased. Both of these are in the direction hypothesized by the investigators.
3. a.   180 dyads were involved in the predischarge interviews which would be 360 individuals; I calculate 153 dyads across the 4 cohorts at 2 weeks postdischarge which would be 306 of the original 360. (The text of the article states that there were 158 dyads that completed both the predischarge and the 2-week postdischarge interviews. I cannot find an explanation or source for this discrepancy. 140 dyads completed all three of the data collection phases, which would be 280 individuals out of the original 360 individuals.)
    b.   Caregivers were the subjects in Table 4.
    c.   There was a statistically significant difference between the intervention group and the control groups with the intervention group scoring higher on the continuity of information variable at 2 months postdischarge.

CHAPTER 19

Numbers in parentheses refer to the relevant chapter in the textbook.

Problem Statement and Purpose (Chapter 3)

1.   Yes, in the second paragraph. (Anger is underexamined in early adolescents.)
2.   Yes, in the first paragraph.
3.   Yes
4.   Yes
5.   Yes
6.   Yes

7. I would have liked a bit more of an explanation as to why this area was considered significant by the investigators. I have a background in adolescent psych so I could develop an argument for significance, but I don't know if my explanation is the same as the researchers.
8. Given the intent of the study, i.e. explication of a model, there was little discussion of the pragmatics associated with completing the study.
9. The statement of purpose is the last sentence of the second paragraph. "To examine symptom patterns and diminished general well-being as negative outcomes of trait and state anger and to examine vigor and change as positive outcomes of trait and state anger in early adolescents" (p. 470).

The Hypotheses (Chapter 3)
1. Yes, all hypotheses are related to the research's purpose.
2. Yes, all hypotheses were stated in a declarative form. They were not easy to find, simply because they were incorporated into the conceptual narrative.
3. Yes, both types of variables were identified.
4. Yes. It may not be immediately obvious that the variables are measurable. They are complex variables and will not be easy to measure.
5. Yes
6. Yes
7. Yes
8. Yes
9. Yes
10. Yes, for most of the hypotheses. Those that dealt with the indirect relationships among variables were not as clearly explained as the more direct relationships.
11. Not applicable

Review of Literature (Chapter 4)
1. The gap existed between the literature that identified anger as a major concern in early adolescence AND minimal literature describing either positive or negative outcomes related to anger.
2. Yes. This section of the report is a clear example of critical thinking because the investigators are spelling out their thinking about the relationship among the variables.
3. Yes, although I think an additional paragraph that addressed how anger is a major concern in early adolescence would have been helpful.
4. No. It is possible that there are no studies that address anger in early adolescence. The literature that was reported was much more theoretical which did fit as the investigators were examining the variables from a theoretical perspective.
5. Studies were not critiqued.
6. No, appeared to be conceptual literature only.
7. Yes
8. No, areas relevant to each hypothesis were summarized but there was no overall summary.
9. There was no synthesis summary.
10. The organization of the review of literature was appropriate for the type of study. The study was focused more on an understanding of theoretical relationships of the variables in a particular population. The need was one of understanding a body of literature in relation to a group that had not been addressed previously.

11. Yes

Theoretical Framework (Chapter 5)

1. Yes. The theoretical framework was built around Spielberger's conception of trait anger and state anger and the relationship between these two components of anger and two positive outcomes (vigor and change) and two negative outcomes (symptom pattern and diminished well-being).
2. The connection between the study of anger in early adolescence and nursing was not explicitly addressed.
3. Yes
4. Yes. I had the sense that the theoretical material had been cut in the interest of article space. I have spent some time working with the variables in the study so had little difficulty in being able to see the links among them. I am not sure how easily the links would be understood by a novice reader. This will have to be your call.
5. Yes
6. Yes
7. Yes

Chapters 6, 7, and 8 are not relevant to this study

Research Design (Chapter 9)

1. Yes
2. Yes, very little control required given the nature of the study.
3. Yes
4. Yes
5. Selection bias would the greatest threat to internal validity. There was little discussion of the degree of population representation present in the sample.
6. None
7. Selection effects would the greatest threat to external validity.
8. None, and given the nature of the study, there would have been very little that could have been done in this area. The discussion of the findings were limited as they should have been.

Experimental and Quasiexperimental Designs (Chapter 10)

Not applicable since this was neither an experimental nor a quasiexperimental design.

Nonexperimental Designs (Chapter 11)

1. This study fits in that group of studies labeled "causal modeling." The study design would be labeled "descriptive" or "exploratory" if we limited ourselves to the traditional conceptions of experimental research. This study is addressing the relationship among variables that would lay the groundwork for testing predictive statements.
2. Yes
3. It is trying to understand a series of relationships among variables in a population that has not been previously studied.
4. Yes
5. Yes
6. Yes
7. Comes close in a couple of areas but does not really go beyond the data in the study.

8. No
9. Not appropriate
10. Discussed in the findings area and in the suggestions for future research.

Sampling (Chapter 12)

1. Yes
2. Yes, if we consider all seventh and eighth graders as the population. The question that would need to be addressed is the definition of early adolescence as between 12 and 14 years of age but limiting the study to seventh and eighth graders. There will be a large group of sixth graders who are 12 and another large group of 14 year olds who will be ninth graders.
3. See comment in #2 above
4. Yes
5. Were not discussed
6. Probably
7. Convenience sample. Yes
8. Selection bias — unclear about how the sample represents the population
9. The investigators told us that the sample size was appropriate for the LISREL equation.
10. Yes
11. Yes
12. Yes

Legal and Ethical Issues (Chapter 13)

1. Yes
2. Yes. Packets of information were sent home with the students. Students had to have their parents' consent and each student consented to participate.
3. Yes
4. Yes
5. Is not explicitly stated but since there was a consent form and the study had been approved by a university IRB I would think that the risks had been explained.
6. Yes
7. No
8. The maintenance of data was not discussed. Students completed the survey forms in an auditorium setting so individuals could know who participated and who did not, but there is no reason to suspect that they had access to each other's data.

Data Collection Methods (Chapter 14)

1. Yes
2. Yes
3. Yes
4. The study was not a clinical setting, but the methods used were appropriate for the study.
5. Yes

The specific areas of data collection methods listed were not relevant for this particular study.

Reliability and Validity (Chapter 15)

1. Yes
2. Yes

3. Yes
4. Yes, from the information given these are instruments that have been well-tested.
5. Not applicable
6. Yes
7. Yes

Descriptive Data Analysis (Chapter 16)
1. Yes
2. All data were treated as interval data.
3. Yes
4. Means, standard deviations, and ranges for the study variables. Demographic characteristics of the sample.
5. Yes
6. Yes
7. Yes
8. Yes
9. Agree with the text and extend it

Inferential Data Analysis (Chapter 17)
1. No
2. Interval
3. Yes
4. Yes
5. Yes
6. Yes
7. Yes
8. Yes
9. Yes, if one has spent some effort in studying the statistical procedure used. The intent of the testing and use of this procedure can be intuitively determined, but it requires some study to understand what the technique accomplishes.
10. No
11. Not applicable

Analysis of Findings (Chapter 18)
1. Yes
2. Yes
3. Yes
4. Yes
5. Yes, in some respects the figures of the models are repetitive but the diagrams help in visualizing the relationships.
6. Yes
7. Yes
8. Not applicable
9. There was some mention of how the results might be clinically relevant but it was touched lightly which was appropriate.
10. Generalizations were not made which was appropriate.
11. Yes

CHAPTER 20

Activity 1
1. Florence Nightingale
2. B, D, A, E, C
3. Problem = something from clinical experience/practice triggers the hunt for a solution; Knowledge = ideas generated by reading articles, attending conferences
4. 8, 9, 1, 5, 7, 11, 2, 10, 6, 3, 4
5. Positive attitude and commitment by clinicians involved; combined effort of relevant clinicians, experts, opinion leaders, and administration in the process; evaluation of both the process and the outcome.

Activity 2
There is no specific answer for this activity. Your instructor will probably use the topics you have developed in a class discussion of how nurses can move from the literature to practice OR how we can move from no literature to creating some literature.

Activity 3
Again, there is no specific answer.

Activity 4
1. a = c; with other evidence could be decision driven
    b = c
    c = c
    d = c
2. a. Bull, Hansen, and Gross   (Discharge planning for elders & caregivers)
        Cohen and Levy   (Response to bone marrow transplant)
        Mahon, Yarcheski, and Yarcheski   (Outcomes of anger in early adolescence)
        LoBiondo-Wood et al.   (Family pretransplant response to child's transplant)

b, c, d, and e will have answers specific to your setting and clinical area.

Appendix B
Home Pages

Agency for Health Care Policy and Research

U.S. government site that provides links to research portfolio, guidelines, and medical outcomes, consumer health information, news, resources, and electronic catalog.

URL: http://www.ahcpr.gov/

National Library of Medicine-PubMed

Provides free access to MEDLINE's search service to access 9 million citations.

Searches by terms, authors, or journal titles. Provides sets of related articles precomputed for each article cited.

URL: http://www.ncbi.nlm.nih.gov/PubMed/

Virginia Henderson International Nursing Library

Sigma Theta Tau International's Honor Society of Nursing web site which has links to the Registry of Nursing Research (free to members as of 1/98) and The Online Journal of Knowledge Synthesis (provides a critical review of research pertinent to clinical practice problems) available with a subscription fee.

URL: http://www.stti.iupui.edu/library/